Frontiers in Cancer Immunology
(*Volume 2*)
Systems Biology in Cancer Immunotherapy

Authored By

Mahbuba Rahman
Sidra Medical and Research Center
Doha
Qatar

Frontiers in Cancer Immunology

Frontiers in Cancer Immunology; Systems Biology in Cancer Immunotherapy

Volume # 2

ISSN (Online): 2405-9110

ISSN (Print): 2405-9102

Author: Mahbuba Rahman

ISBN (eBook): 978-1-68108-307-0

ISBN (Print): 978-1-68108-308-7

Reprints and Revisions:

First published in 2016

advertisements or ideas contained in the Work.

Limitation of Liability:

In no event will Bentham Science Publishers, its staff, editors and/or authors, be liable for any damages, including, without limitation, special, incidental and/or consequential damages and/or damages for lost data and/or profits arising out of (whether directly or indirectly) the use or inability to use the Work. The entire liability of Bentham Science Publishers shall be limited to the amount actually paid by you for the Work.

General:

1. Any dispute or claim arising out of or in connection with this License Agreement or the Work (including non-contractual disputes or claims) will be governed by and construed in accordance with the laws of the U.A.E. as applied in the Emirate of Dubai. Each party agrees that the courts of the Emirate of Dubai shall have exclusive jurisdiction to settle any dispute or claim arising out of or in connection with this License Agreement or the Work (including non-contractual disputes or claims).

2. Your rights under this License Agreement will automatically terminate without notice and without the need for a court order if at any point you breach any terms of this License Agreement. In no event will any delay or failure by Bentham Science Publishers in enforcing your compliance with this License Agreement constitute a waiver of any of its rights.

3. You acknowledge that you have read this License Agreement, and agree to be bound by its terms and conditions. To the extent that any other terms and conditions presented on any website of Bentham Science Publishers conflict with, or are inconsistent with, the terms and conditions set out in this License Agreement, you acknowledge that the terms and conditions set out in this License Agreement shall prevail.

Bentham Science Publishers Ltd.
Executive Suite Y - 2
PO Box 7917, Saif Zone
Sharjah, U.A.E.
Email: subscriptions@benthamscience.org

BENTHAM SCIENCE

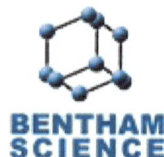

CONTENTS

FOREWORD

I am honoured to be able to contribute to this exciting eBook about Systems Biology in Cancer Immunotherapy. The eBook has excellent credentials for describing important knowledge and approaches for the understanding of cancer cell metabolism and immunotherapy.

Dr. Mahbuba Rahman is one of my former PhD students, and she is among the top students in our laboratory in Kyushu Institute of Technology. She has long been involved in cancer research based on molecular biology as well as ^{13}C-metabolic flux analysis. She has published many articles in this area.

In summary, I am delighted to see such expertly produced and well referenced eBook which will contribute to molecular biology, biochemical science, and medical science.

Dr. Kazuyuki Shimizu
Institute of Advanced Biosciences
Keio University
Tsuruoka, Yamagata
Japan

PREFACE

Robustness is an essential property of all biological systems. This property is maintained and controlled by a large number of protein and signalling molecules, enzymes and regulatory molecules, which form an intricate regulatory network to transfer signals inside and outside of the cell. Considering the complex regulatory network of a cell inside its own milieu or its surrounding environment, cells have been referred to as 'systems' for more than a century ago. These networks control several checkpoints that are associated with cell proliferation, differentiation and metabolic regulation. Interestingly, the robustness or plasticity is observed both in healthy cells and in diseased or transformed cells like cancer cells. However, in cancer cells, the checkpoints are either mutated or dysregulated. Therefore, an in-depth understanding of the systems of these cells is an essential requisite prior to developing therapy against cancer. This can be achieved by using robust approach, such as the systems biology approach.

The technological platforms for systems biology are rooted in molecular biology. Unlike the conventional molecular biology techniques, systems biology takes advantage of the high-throughput omics platforms. The main strength of this approach is that it integrates results carried out by researchers of broad disciplinary such as molecular biology, immunology, bioinformatics, physicians and even the R&D of pharmaceutical companies in different parts of the world. Thus the approach produces unbiased data which enables researchers to investigate the system of a cell.

Over the past several years, systems biology approaches have been applied in different areas of life sciences research including cancer. Researchers were able to understand the hallmarks of cancer cells such as abnormal cell growth, inflammation, dysregulated metabolic pathways, drug resistance properties, *etc.* It also enabled researchers to investigate specific fields of cancer immunology including identification of cancer related signature molecule on the immune cells, biomarker identification, effect of monotherapy and combination therapy in tissue culture and mouse model. More recently, systems biology approach has been applied to cancer immunotherapy. Several immunotherapy drugs received US FDA approval and are at phase III of clinical trials. However, many immunotherapy drugs that are tested in laboratory tissue culture and mouse model failed to show significant tumor regression in patients. Investigation of the underlying cause of therapy resistance at the genetic and phenotypic level requires the use of robust approach like systems biology. Although systems biology is still at its infancy in cancer immunotherapy research, considering the strength of the approach to dissect a robust system or cell, in this volume of eBook series, we discussed the scope of systems biology in cancer. However, during preparation of this volume, an important platform of systems biology, metabolic flux analysis (MFA) was found to be less studied. This is a robust tool to understand the metabolic concentration of a cell resulting from specific cellular processes and from the function of a gene. Future research in cancer immunotherapy should consider implementing this method to understand and tie the diseased phenotype with the targeted cells.

Dr. Mahbuba Rahman
Sidra Medical and Research Center
Doha
Qatar
Email: mrahman1@sidra.org

CHAPTER 1

Immune System in Cancer

Abstract: Our immune system is a dynamic environment that is orchestrated by a network of immune cells and signalling molecules and is differentially expressed and regulated at different stages of life. Interestingly, components of the immune system function differently under diseased or non-diseased state, healthy or immune-deficient state. Cancer is generally regarded as a genetic disease and caused from inflammation. Due to the complex nature of the disease, it is necessary to understand how the immune system responses in a tumor environment. A detailed understanding on the cancer immuno-biology will enable formulation of appropriate treatment strategies for cancer.

Keywords: Circulating tumor cells, Cytokines, Dendritic cells, Immuno-escape, Immune-surveillance, Immuno-system, Regulatory T cells, Tumor associated antigens, Tumor derived factors, Tumor specific antigens.

INTRODUCTION

Cancer is a multistage disease that progresses *via* prolonged accumulation of multiple genetic and/or epigenetic changes which control cell proliferation, survival, differentiation, migration and interactions with neighbouring cells and stroma. More than 200 different types of cancers have been reported. The classification of cancer is based on the tissue of origin or pathogenesis (Table **1**). Classification based on tissue of origin shows that cancer can originate from any tissues of the body and can be either localized or systemic. Whatever the origin of cancer is, our immune system, which is our body's defensive system, responds to the inflammations caused during cancer development [1, 2].

In general, our immune system performs two critical activities in response to exposure to foreign particles: 'recognition' where the cells identifies the harmful agent called 'antigen' and 'effector responses' by which specific receptors

Mahbuba Rahman

expressed on the surface of immune cells bind antigens and confer protection by cellular behaviors. In case of cancer, where the cancer cells originate from the host's body, cells of both the innate immune system and the adaptive immune system are often involved [3, 4].

Table 1. Classification of cancer based on tissue of origin and pathological point of view [5].

Type of cancer	Tissue of Origin	Special features
Carcinoma	Originate from epithelial cells in skin or tissues that line or cover internal organs. About 80% human cancers are of this type.	Localized, also known as solid tumor. The tumor is often confined by basement membrane. Until the tumor cells turn into invasive carcinomas where the basement membrane is disrupted and tumor grows into the surrounding tissues.
Sarcoma	Originate in bone, cartilage, fat, muscle, blood vessels and other connective or supportive tissues.	Also known as solid tumor
Leukemia	Originate in blood-forming tissues such as bone marrow and causes large number of abnormal blood cells to be produced and enter the bloodstream.	Systemic and also known as liquid tumor.
Lymphoma	Originate in the cells of the immune system.	Known as liquid tumor

BASICS OF THE HUMAN IMMUNO SYSTEM

Our immune system broadly comprises of two major subgroups: the innate/acquired immune system and the adaptive immune system. The primary function of the innate system is to provide a rapid non-specific response to foreign invaders such as virus, bacteria or foreign antigens, wound, inflammatory insult or newly initiated diseased cells. On the other hand, the adaptive immune system helps to provide a latent but highly specific response by producing antibodies against foreign or non-self antigens to generate immune memory against the antigens that cross the first line of the defensive system. Hence, the immune system plays crucial role to protect the body from infection. Each of the arms of the immune system consists of cellular and humoral (antibody) components which function in unique ways to combat against the infection. Despite the uniqueness, there is interplay between components of the systems that protects the body from foreign invaders [6].

The major difference between the innate/acquired immunity and the adaptive immunity is that innate immune response are non-specific and occurs within minutes and lasts for a few days whereas, the adaptive immunity occurs over weeks to years and is more specific where the immunological memory invokes rapid eradication of subsequent infections. This mechanism of the adaptive system is used as the basis for immunization and vaccination in humans. Despite these differences, the main function of the immune system is self-nonself discrimination including the foreign invaders and modified or altered cells (*e.g.*, cancer or malignant cells) to protect the organism from foreign invaders or eliminate abnormal cells. To perform this, both the adaptive and innate immune system connects in some way with the help of the cells of the system and specific molecules to initiate acute inflammation followed by wound healing of the diseased cells [7].

Origin and Formation of the Immune System

Our immune system comprises of a varied collection of interconnected cells and tissues that are distributed throughout the body. The lymphoid organs that consist of the primary lymphoid organ (*e.g.*, bone marrow and thymus) and the secondary lymphoid organ (*e.g.*, regional lymph nodes and spleen) are connected to one another through two separate circulatory systems. These are the blood system and the lymphatic system. White blood cells are produced and differentiated in the primary lymphoid organs. The secondary lymphoid organs together with the circulatory systems outside of the primary lymphoid organs are collectively referred to as the "periphery." While the lymph nodes and spleen serve to filter and trap foreign molecules and cells that are delivered from the tissues *via* the lymph fluid or the blood, the secondary lymphoid organs provide organized tissues in which the white blood cells can encounter foreign antigen molecules and physically interact with other white blood cells to initiate an appropriate response [8].

The majority of the cells of the immune system are circulatory or migratory. All cells of the immune system originate from the bone-marrow hematopoietic stem cells (HSCs). These multipotent stem cells differentiate into myeloid and lymphoid progenitors. The myeloid progenitors subsequently generate megakaryotes, erythrocytes, mast cells, macrophages, dendritic cells (DCs), neutrophils, basophils, and eosinophils and the lymphoid progenitors give rise to small lymphocytes (B- and T cells) and large granular lymphocytes (natural killer (NK) cells). Overall, the cells of the immune system can be grouped into three major categories: the lymphocytes (*e.g.*, T cells, B cells and natural killer (NK) cells), the myeloid cells (*e.g.*, the antigen presenting cells (APCs) such as macrophages and dendritic cells (DCs); and the granulocytic cells (*e.g.*, neutrophils, basophils and eosinophils) [8].

Among the myeloid progenitors, mast cells, macrophages, dendritic cells, neutrophils, basophils, and eosinophils and the NK cells of the lymphoid progenitor are the cells of the innate immune system. On the other hand, the lymphoid progenitors or B and T lymphocytes are the cells of the adaptive immune system and produce stronger effect and create immunological memory where the signature antigen of each pathogen is stored in specific lymphocytes (also known as clones).

Some of the precursor T cells require migration to the thymus for differentiation into two distinct types of T cells, the CD4+ T helper cell and the CD8+ pre-cytotoxic T cell. In the thymus, two types of T helper cells are produced, Th1 cells and Th2 cells. The Th1 cells help CD8+ pre-cytotoxic T cells to differentiate into cytotoxic T cells, and Th2 cells help B cells to differentiate into plasma cells that secrete antibodies [9].

CANCER IMMUNOLOGY

Cancer is a multi-factorial genetic disease. Although treatment modalities are available for cancer, the cure rate is not satisfactory for all the different types of cancer mentioned earlier in Table **1**. Many cancers are not even clinically apparent and in many case prognosis may be poor. Therefore prevention from cancer might be a more acceptable strategy to treat cancer. Cancer can be considered as inflammation of normal cells. Since our immune system plays crucial role in responding to infection, knowledge on cancer immunology can play dual role such as in identifying cancer biomarkers by measuring different components of the immune system that we mentioned earlier and also use the information for therapeutic purposes. In this respect, active cancer immuno-therapy or cancer vaccines can be preventive or therapeutic. A detailed understanding on this mechanism requires a basic understanding of how the immune system responds to tumor. Recent studies show that our immune system recognizes tumor specific antigens and possess anti-tumor activity. This process is now well known as immune-surveillance. However, tumor cells can also escape the immune system and lead to tumor progression in a process called immune-escape. We will discuss both the mechanisms to understand tumor or cancer immunology [6].

IMMUNO-SURVEILLANCE

Most of the cancer is caused from inflammation. However, our immune system plays three primary roles in the prevention of tumors. These are: (i) immune cells protect the host from virus-induced tumors by eliminating or suppressing viral infections, (ii) timely eliminates pathogens and resolute inflammation to prevent the establishment of an inflammatory environment which is the primary cause of many tumorigenesis, and (iii) the immune system specifically identify and eliminate tumor cells on the basis of their expression of tumor-specific antigens or molecules induced by cellular stress. Both the innate immune system and the adaptive immune system take part in this process. The antitumor immunity is mediated by cytotoxic T cells (CTLs), natural killer (NK) and natural killer T (NKT) cells. Of these, cytotoxic T cells (CTLs), or more specifically CD8+ T cells are of the adaptive immune system. NK cells, NKT and γδT are effector cells of the innate immune system. Dendritic cells (DCs) play important role as antigen presenting cell and co-ordinates the activities of the anti –tumor responses. The other cells such as tumor associated macrophages (TAM), T regulatory cells (Treg), and myeloid- derived suppressor cells (MDSCs) form immune-suppressive network [10].

Innate Immune System in Antitumor Response

Natural Killer (NK) Cells

Natural killer (NK) cells play key role in innate anti-tumor response. They perform this by employing several effector mechanisms including perforin, death receptor ligands, and interferon-gamma (IFN-γ). NK cells have the ability to lyse MHC class I deficient tumors without prior stimulation. However, in the tumor microenvironment, its function is regulated through a combination of inhibitory and activating receptors, cytokines (*e.g.*, IL-2 and IL-15), and by co-stimulatory molecules including CD80, CD86, CD40, CD70 and ICOS [11].

NK cells express different types of inhibitory receptors. These receptors deliver negative regulatory signals following engagement with target cell MHC class I molecules. The inhibitory molecules include killer cell immunoglobulin-like receptors (KIRs) and the C-type lectin-like molecules (CD94 and NKG2A/E) in primates. Individual NK cells display varying pattern of the inhibitory proteins which allows an increased ability of the NK population to detect losses of individual MHC class I alleles [11]. NK cells express several families of activating receptors including the natural cytotoxicity receptors (NKp46, NKp44, NKp30 and NKp80), additional Ly49 proteins and NKG2D. NKG2D ligands include the MHC lass I related molecules MICA and MICB and six UL16 binding proteins in humans and the retinoic acid- early inducible gene products (RIG) are induced by DNA damages through the pathway that involves ATM, ATR, Chk-1 and Chk-2. The surface activation of these ligands on stressed cells triggers NKG2D dependent activation of NK, NKT, γδ T and CD8 T cells, leading to inhibition of tumor growth [11].

Macrophages

Macrophages are required for homeostatic clearance of apoptotic cells, control of epithelial cell turnover, and assist tissues in the adaptation to stress conditions [12]. Macrophages play diverse role in tumor suppression. Necrotic tumor cells release stress induced molecules such as HSP-70 or HMGB1 which may trigger TLR- dependent macrophage activation and produces cytotoxic reactive oxygen and nitrogen species and secrets inflammatory cytokines.

However, macrophages can also contribute to tumor protection and tumor progression. In tumor microenvironment, particular type of macrophages are present and these are known as tumor associated macrophages (TAMs) (Fig. **1**). They may stimulate antitumor T cells while suppressing CD4+CD25+ regulatory T cells (Tregs) through IL-6 release [12]. Tumor cells exploit macrophage activities which is critical for wound healing. This breaks down the basement membranes and establishes robust vascular network, driving tumor cell invasion, expansion and metastasis [13, 14].

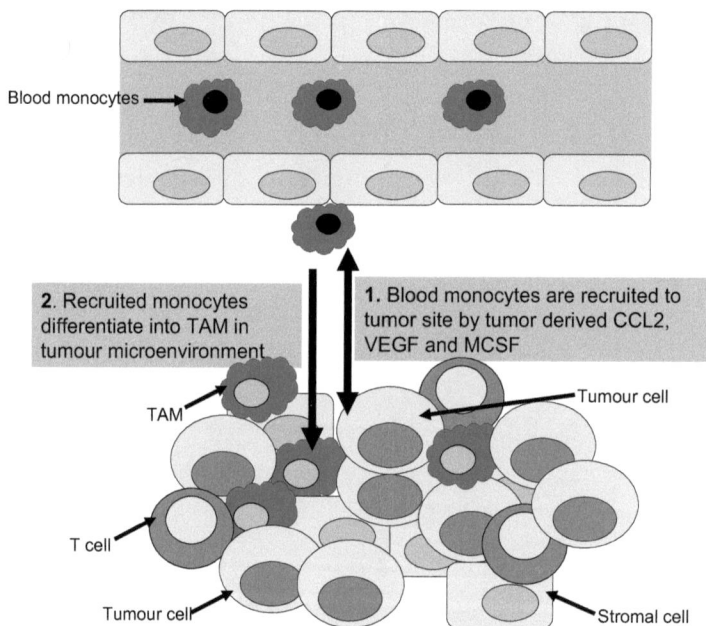

Fig. (1). Tumor associated macrophages (TAM) in solid-tumor environment (Modified from Mantovani *et al.*, 2007).

Dendritic Cells

Dendritic cells are antigen presenting cells (APCs) and they also play role in processing and presenting the tumor associated antigens. In human, multiple DC subsets exist. They vary in location, phenotype and perform specialised function. DCs are classified as conventional DC (cDC), plasmacytoid DC (pDC) and inflammatory monocyte-derived (Mo) DC. The cDC are further divided into lymphoid-resident and migratory DC. This classification is based on the location of the lymphocyte. While the lymphoid resident DC capture antigen (Ag) directly from the blood, lymph and other DCs, the migratory DC reside in the peripheral organs such as lung, skin and gut. These DCs capture antigen from the periphery organ and then migrate to lymphoid tissues where they present Ag directly to T cells, or share Ag with lymphoid resident DC. In both locations, cDCs further segregate into multiple subsets with significant functional specialization. While we already discussed how the DC helps in immune- protection, the particular type of DC associated with anti-tumor response is IFN- producing killer dendritic cells (IKDC). These cells express some of the NK cell, produce type I interferons and are cytotoxic. The phenotype of these cell is distinct from NK cells and plasmacytoid dendritic cells. IKDCs may be activated with NKG2D ligands and lyse tumor targets through TRAIL. Following migration to draining lymph nodes, IKDCs display antigen- presenting cell features which includes upregulation of MHC and co-stimulatory molecules and stimulation of T-cell response [15].

NKT Cells

NKT cells express an invariant T-cell receptor alpha chain and NK-cell markers CD161 or NKR-P1. The invariant T-cell receptors are specific for glycolipid antigens presented by CD1d which is an MHC class I related molecule expressed on antigen-presenting cells (APC) and some cancer cells. Depending on the mode of activation, NKT cells produce both Th1 and Th2 cytokines, which play key regulatory roles for the cytokine milieu and glycolipid antigen repertoire present in the tumor microenvironment. NKTcell mediated tumor destruction involves IFN-γ production followed by activation of NK cells and CD8+ T-cells to exert cytotoxic activity. In addition, NKT cells are also required for the therapeutic effects of GM-CSF and IL- 12 based cytokine strategies [11].

$\gamma\delta T$ cells

These are small population of T lymphocytes which shows an integrated role of innate and adaptive immunity. $\gamma\delta$T cells undergo VDJ recombination during thymic development, although their TCR diversity is relatively limited compared to conventional $\alpha\beta$T cells. $\gamma\delta$T cells function more in pattern recognition. These cells constitute a significant proportion of intraepithelial lymphocytes (IEL) in the skin, gastrointestinal mucosa and genitourinary tract mucosa. γδ T cells recognize unique ligands expressed by tumors that are not recognized by αβT cells.

γδ T cells also serve as the major early source of IFN-γ during disease development and mediates direct antitumor cytotoxicity. IL-17 secreting γδT cells (Vδ4/Vδ6) showed early trafficking to tumors following chemotherapy administration [16].

Granulocytes

Like macrophages, granulocytes have complex interaction with tumors. In the context of its role in tumor suppression, granulocytes may contribute to tumor destruction through the release of toxic moieties packaged in granules, generation of reactive oxygen species, and secretion of inflammatory cytokines. Experimental tumors engineered to secret granulocyte-colony stimulating factors (GCSF) stimulated the adaptive T- cell responses that eradicated subsequent tumor challenges [16]. Neutrophils also play role to generate antitumor effects of Her-2/neu-based DNA vaccinations in a transgenic breast cancer model[16].

Adaptive Immune System in Anti-tumor Response

B Lymphocytes

B lymphocytes constitute a major class of the adaptive immune system. B cells are small circulating lymphocytes and are distinguishable by the surface expression of a B cell specific form of the CD45 protein. This variant is called B220 and it serves as a pan-B cell marker. There are two distinct type of B cell subsets: the B1B cells and the B2B cells. B1 cells express low levels of B 220 and many of them express CD5 surface markers. The B1 populations are long-lived and self-renewing lymphocytes and they reside primarily in the peritoneal and pleural cavities. On the other hand, majority of the B cells fall into B2B cell category. These are called conventional B cells and they express high levels of B220. In addition to these surface markers, all B cells also express antigen receptors or antibodies (also known as immunoglobulins) on their surface and are capable of recognizing antigen without the involvement of other components of the immune system. Each antibody molecule comprises of two chains, a light chain (L) and a heavy chain [17, 18].

T Lymphocytes

There are several types of T lymphocytes of which the majority are helper T cell, killer T cell and regulatory T cells (Treg). Their classification is based on the presence of the T cell receptors (TCR) or cell surface markers such as CD4+, CD8+ *etc.* Unlike the B cells, which comprise a single major lineage, there are a number of specialized T cell population that are phenotypically and functionally distinguished by the presence of a particular surface marker, CD3. While B220 is the marker for all cells of the B cell lineage, CD3, a complex comprised of multiple surface glycoproteins is considered a pan-T-cell marker [9, 17].

Early progenitor T cells are derived in tissue of general hematopoiesis, such as in the bone marrow, and then migrate to the thymus to develop. Immunocompetent T cells then exit the thymus. T lymphocytes that originate from lymphoid organs and matures in the thymus are generally known as helper T cell (Th). The CD4+ T helper cells are classified into two major groups, Th1 and Th2. Th1 cells express interferon (IFN)-γ and controls cellular immunity. The Th2 cells on the other hand produce interleukin (IL)-4, IL-5 and IL-13 and regulate humoral immunity [19].

Another subset of T helper cell is Th17 which produces IL-17A, IL-17F and IL-6 are known as pro-inflammatory. They respond to immune defense against extracellular bacteria [19].

Another type of T cell is killer T cell or CD8$^+$ T cell. These are also known as cytotoxic T lymphocytes (CTLs). CD8$^+$ T cells recognize and kill virus infected cells or cancerous cells. These cells are specific to MHC class I molecules and kill their targets by inducing a programmed cell death (PCD) response in the infected cells [19].

The other class of T cell is regulatory T (Treg) cells. These are heterogeneous population of T cells that play crucial roles in maintaining the immune homeostasis. The CD4+CD25+Foxp3+ 'naturally occurring' Treg (nTreg) cells are generated in the thymus. Another Treg cell is CD4+CD25+Foxp3 induced' Treg (iTreg) cells. These are generated in peripheral lymphoid organs. However, these can be produced in cultures following stimulation with antigens and Treg-inducing cytokines such as transforming growth factor (TGF)-β. Foxp3+ protein is the most distinct marker for nTreg and iTreg cells and also crucial for their function and activation [19].

Both the B lymphocytes and the T lymphocytes of the adaptive immune system use complex genetic machinery for the construction of antigen specific receptors. The receptors comprises of two subunits, one requiring the assembly of V, D, J DNA elements and the other subunit requires the V and J elements. Random pairing of the rearranged VDJ- and VJ-bearing products yields a large amount of combinatorial variability and increases diversity at the DNA level. For example, at the junction of the newly combined elements (D to J, V to DJ, and V to J) nucleotides may be added or deleted. This will alter the amino acid sequence of the receptors. The segments of the polypeptide chain display maximum diversity and correspond to the regions of the folded receptor that most intimately contact antigen [1].

Mechanism of Antitumor T-cell Response

The principal mechanism involved in the priming of anti-tumor T cells is associated with the presentation of tumor associated antigens by professional APCs such as the dendritic cell (DC). Tumor associated antigens and their epitopes are an important area for clinical cancer immunotherapy. These can be used for two major purposes, (i) development of the active immunotherapy and (ii) development of passive immunotherapy. The active immunotherapy involves antigen-specific vaccination in order to induce and boost the antitumor activity of specific CD4+ and CD8+ T cells within the tumor host. The passive immunotherapy is the adoptive T-cell therapy used for the elimination of cancer cells by antigen-specific, ex-vivo expanded and adoptively transferred autologous CTLs [20, 21]. Some of these antigens are discussed below:

Tumor Specific (TSA) and Tumor Associated Antigens (TAA)

Tumors express many molecules or antigens that are recognized by the immune system. These antigens are broadly classified as tumor specific antigens (TSA) and tumor associated antigens (TAA). TSA antigens are expressed only on tumors whereas tumor associated antigens are expressed on both tumors and normal cells, with some important differences [21].

Tumor specific antigens are classified into five groups: antigens resulting from mutations, antigens encoded by cancer-germline genes, viral antigens, differentiation antigens and over-expressed antigens [21].

Antigens Resulting from Mutation

Antigens among this group show nonsynonymous somatic base substitutions in ubiquitously expressed protein-coding sequences. This type of mutations are a frequent source of tumor-specific antigenic peptides that are recognized by T cells. The amino acid encoded by the mutated codon either enable a peptide to bind to an HLA molecule or modifies the shape of an HLA-binding peptide so that new T cell receptors (TCRs) recognize it like a new epitope. Mutations may be caused by chemical or physical carcinogens, random mutations, or non-random mutations in the cancer related genes mentioned in Table 2. Although the mutation is present within the DNA sequence encoding the peptide, somatic mutations can also be caused through frameshift mutations. The mutated antigens have several important advantages for cancer vaccines as these antigens are truly tumor specific and do not induce T cell tolerance. In addition, T cells that recognize these antigens do not recognize any normal cell [21]. Some mentionable "antigenic" mutated oncogenes include CDK4, N- ras, B-raf, BCR-ABL, P53 *etc.* [22].

Antigens Encoded by Cancer-germline Genes

These are known as 'shared antigens' because they are encoded by the cancer-germline genes and these are expressed in various proportions in different tumors. The genes belonging to this group include MAGE-A, MAGE-B, MAGE-C, LAGE/NY-ESO-1 and SSX (Table 2). Cancer- germline gene expression depends on the hypomethylation of their promoters and their expression correlates with genome-wide demethylation. As a result, many tumors often co-express several cancer-germline genes, while some express none of them [22].

Table 2. Different classes of tumor specific (TSA) and tumor associated antigens (TAA) [5, 24].

Classes of Tumor Antigen	Gene/protein	Type of Cancer
Tumor antigens resulting from mutations		
	Alpha-actinin 4	Lung carcinoma
	ARTC1	Melanoma
	BCR-ABL fusion protein	Chronic myeloid leukemia
	B-RAF	Melanoma
	CASP-5	Colorectal, gastric and endometrial carcinoma
	CASP-8	Head and neck squamous cell carcinoma
	Beta-catenin/Cadherin-associated protein	Melanoma
	Cdc27	Melanoma
	CDK4	Melanoma
	CDKN2A	Melanoma
	CLPP	Melanoma
	COA-1	Colorectal carcinoma
	EFTUD2	Melanoma
	Elongation factor 2	lung squamous CC
	Hsp70-2	Renal cell carcinoma
	MUM-1	Melanoma
	Neo-PAP	Melanoma
	NFYC	Lung squamous cell carcinoma
	P53	Head and neck squamous cell carcinoma
	K-ras	Pancreatic carcinoma
	TGF-betaRII	Colorectal carcinoma
	Triphosphate isomerase	Melanoma

(Table 2) contd.....

Classes of Tumor Antigen	Gene/protein	Type of Cancer
Shared tumor-specific antigens		
	Cyclin-A1	Male germ cell tumor and acute myeloid leukemia.
	Gp100	Melanoma
	MAGE-A1	Melanoma and colorectal carcinoma.
	MAGE-A2	Oral squamous cell carcinoma
	MAGE-A3	Melanoma, cholangiocarcinoma and non-small cell lung carcinoma (NSCLC).
	MAGE-A4	Melanoma and pancreatic cancer.
	MAGE-A6	Melanoma and osseous dysplasia.
	MAGE-A9	Termina osseous dysplasia.
	MAGE-B	Melanoma
	MAGE-C1	Melanoma
	MAGE-C2	Hepatocellular carcinoma and liver cancer.
	GAGE	Melanoma, lung carcinoma, head and neck squamous cell carcinoma, esophageal squamous cell carcinoma, bladder carcinoma *etc.*
	BAGE-1	Chronic lymphocytic leukemia and melanoma.
	LAGE-1	Melanoma and prostate cancer.
	LAGE-2/ NY-ESO-1	Esophageal squamous cell carcinoma and biphasic synovial sarcoma.
	SSX-2	Spindle cell synovial sarcoma and kidney hemangiopericytoma.
	TRAG-3	Lung adenocarcinoma and esophageal cancer.
	XAGE1b/GAGED2A	Non-small cell lung carcinoma (NSCLC) and lung adenocarcinoma.
Differentiation antigens		
	Melan-A/MART-1	Melanoma
	TRP-1	Melanoma
	Tyrosinase	Melanoma

(Table 2) contd.....

Classes of Tumor Antigen	Gene/protein	Type of Cancer
Antigens over-expressed in tumors		
	Adipophilin/ADFP	Lipid-rich carcinoma and kidney cancer.
	ALDH1A1	Gallbladder adenocarcinoma
	BCL-XL	Colorectal cancer and myeloma.
	CD274	Primary mediastinal large B-cell lymphoma
	CD45	Testicular lymphoma
	Cyclin D1	Superficial urinary bladder cancer and breast papillary carcinoma.
	DKK1	Multiple myeloma and myeloma.
	EpCAM	Intestinal epithelial dysplasia.
	EPHA3	Pleomorphic rhabdomyosarcoma and colorectal cancer.
	FGF5 (fibroblast growth factor)	Kaposi's sarcoma.
	G250/MN/CAIX (Carbonic anhydrase IX)	Renal cell carcinoma and clear cell renal carcinoma.
	HER-2/neu	Breast scirrhous carcinoma and lipid rich carcinoma.
	Hepsin	Prostate cancer and ovarian cancer.
	Alpha-fetoprotein	Germ cell tumors and endodermal sinus tumor
	Kalikrein 4	Prostate and ovarian cancer
	Lengsin	Tenosynovial giant cell tumor
	MCSF (macrophage colony-stimulating factor)	Tenosynovial giant cell tumor
	MMP-7	Thymic epithelial tumor
	MUC1	Nodular hidradenoma
	MUC5AC	Anal canal adenocarcinoma and pancreatic cancer.
	Survivin	Cervical carcinosarcoma and ovarian serous cystadenocarcinoma

Viral Antigens

Approximately 20% of global cancer incidence is linked to infectious agents. Of the different types of infectious agents, oncogenic viruses are a source of tumor-specific antigenic peptides. Oncogenic viruses such as antigens derived from the human papiloma virus (E6 and E7 of HPV-16), cervical cancer, those derived from hepatitis B and C virus, those expressed on liver cancers, nasopharyngeal carcinoma antigens encoded by the Epstein-Barr virus proteins LMP1 and LMP2 are some of the example of viral antigens [22].

Differentiation Antigens

These antigens are expressed both in the malignant form of cells and the normal cells of the same lineage. Some mentionable antigens of this class are melanoma differentiation antigens (MDA), circulating carcinoembryonic antigen (CEA) in case of gut carcinoma and prostate specific antigen (PSA) in prostate cancer. However, targeting the differentiation antigens at clinical trial level showed induction of autoimmunity [21].

Over-expressed Antigens

Over-expressed antigens are present in normal cells but these are present at higher levels in tumor cells. MUC1 is one of the first recognized tumor associated antigen which is heavily glycosylated transmembrane protein expressed primarily on polarized ductal or surface epithelia in many organs. MUC1 is highly over-expressed and hypoglycosylated in transformed epithelial cells giving rise to adenocarcinomas of the breast, ovary, lung, prostate, colon, pancreas, *etc.* [22, 23].

Regulatory T Cells in Antitumor Response

Regulatory T cells (Treg) are involved in the maintenance of tolerance and exert immunosuppression depending on the relative number of CD4$^+$ T cells. Unique feature of these cells is that they actively suppress immune response (Fig. **2**). [23]. Treg are classified into two main subsets: the naturally arising Treg (nTreg) and the adaptive Treg (iTreg). The naturally arising Treg develop in the thymus and have high-affinity to TCR triggering suppression of T-cell proliferation. On the other hand, the adaptive Treg develops in the periphery followed by antigenic stimulation in the presence of IL-10 (Tr1 subset) or TGF-beta (Th3 subset). However, phenotypically, both the tregs are indistinsguishible. Thymic development, suboptimal antigenic stimulation and peripheral conversion all contribute to create the total pool of Treg. Their maintenance involves class II

MHC molecules, the cytokine IL-2 and co-stimulatory molecules such as CD28 and CD40. While several molecules have been proposed to identify Treg cells, the actual Treg characterization was the discovery that the forkhead box transcription factor Foxp3 is the master gene of Treg lineage. Very recent studies showed that Foxp3 acts as a mediator that amplifies and fixes pre-established molecular features of Treg cells. However, despite the molecular features of Treg have been extensively dissected, the fine mechanism by which it exerts tumor suppression is not fully resolved yet. This is because Treg cells also inhibits the functions of B lymphocytes, NK cells and dendritic cells [23].

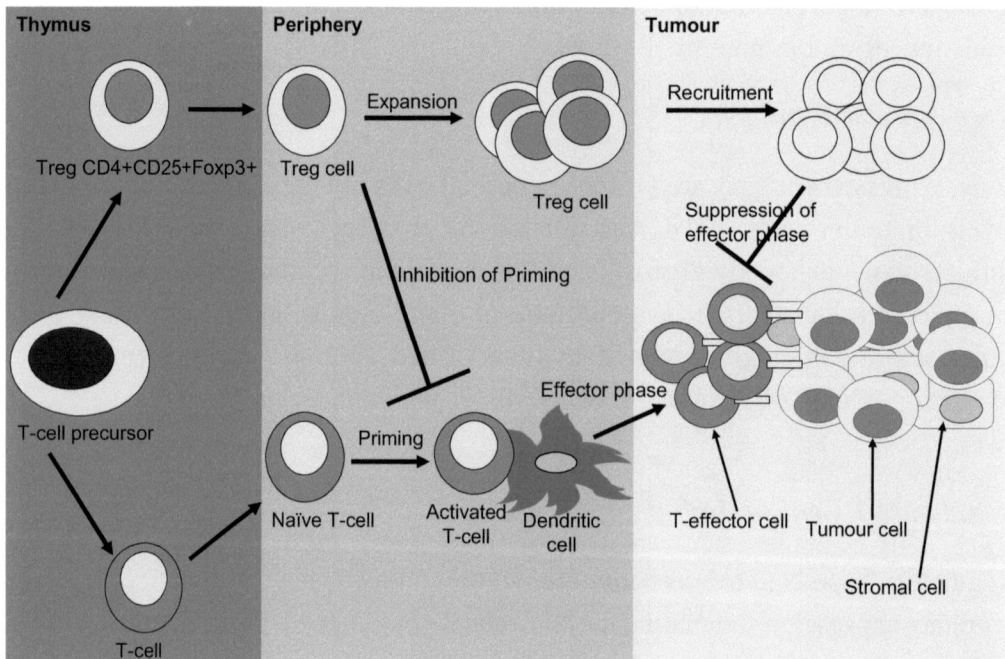

Fig. (2). Immunosuppressive role of Treg cells in tumor environment. (Modified from Piconese and Colombo, 2008).

Natural Killer Cells

NK cells are a third category of T lymphocytes and microscopically distinguished from T and B cells as these lymphocytes are larger and have extensive granules. NK cells account for 5% to 10% of peripheral lymphocytes. NK cells are classified based on the expression of surface markers. All NK cells are recognized by the expression of both CD16 (an Fc receptor molecule) and CD56 (an adhesion molecule). NK-cell populations are further divided based on the differential expression of CD56, where 90% of circulating NK cells express low levels of CD56 while 10% have high levels of CD56 on the cell surface. At a functional level, NK cells with low levels of CD56 show increased cytolytic activity. On the other hand, NK cells with higher CD56 expression levels secret large amounts of a variety of cytokines [23].

NK cells are less specific in contrast to antibody mediated proteins and secret cytotoxins and also participate in Fas-Fas ligand-mediated apoptosis. They perform two major function, (i) kill virus infected cells and tumor cells by secreting cytotoxins, *e.g.*, perforins and granzymes and (ii) produce gamma interferon. Interferons are small proteins that are secreted by the natural killer cells in response to viral infection or double stranded RNAs. Interferons do not directly kill the viral protein, instead they induce the host cell to synthesize non-specific antiviral protein. NK cells are capable of killing with the prior exposure of the virus to the antibody IgG. NK cells also contribute to tumor immunity [23].

Important Cytokines

Full activation, proliferation, and terminal differentiation of lymphocytes depends on several factors including delivery of signals *via* their antigen specific receptor, input from co-stimulatory molecules and exposure to cytokines [1]. Cytokines are non-antibody proteins and they function as mediators and regulators of the two arms of the immune system. Cytokines are produced by both the immune cells and non-immune cells. Naming of cytokines is dependent on the type of cells that produce them. For cxample, 'monokines' are cytokines produced by mononuclear phagocytes; 'lymphokines' are cytokines produced by activated lymphocytes or the Th cells and 'interleukins' are cytokincs that act as mediators between leukocytes [25].

Synthesis of cytokines is initiated by transcription of gene and their mRNAs are short lived and produced as needed for the immune responses. Therefore, cytokines are not stored as pre-formed protein. Generally, cellular response to cytokines is slow (hours) as it requires the synthesis of new mRNA and protein.

Ctokines are pleotropic, *i.e.*, many individual cytokines are produced by many cells types and act on many cell types. In many cases, cytokines have similar actions, and this is due to the nature of the cytokine receptors. Receptors for cytokines are either heterodimers or heterotrimers. These can be grouped into families in which one subunit is common to all members of a given family. The presence of common subunit of the same family can function in binding one cytokine and often respond to another cytokine in the same family. For example, if an individual lacks IL-2, it does not have adverse effect on the person's immune system as other cytokines (IL-15, IL-7, IL-9 *etc.*), assuming its function. Cytokines can also influence the action of other cytokines by acting as antagonistics, additive and synergistic [25].

Cytokines bind to specific receptors on target cells with high affinity. The cells that respond to a cytokine are either: (i) the same cell that secreted the cytokine (autocrine), (ii) a nearby cell (paracrine) or (iii) a distant cell reached through the circulation (endocrine) [25]. Some important cytokines, their function and cell sources are mentioned below:

Mediators of Natural Immunity

Cytokines that belong to this group are tumor necrosis factor alpha (TNF-α), IL-1, IL-10, IL-12, type I interferons (IFN-α and IFN-β), IFN-γ, and chemokines. Of these, TNF-α is produced by activated macrophages in response to lipopolysaccharide (LPS) of Gram negative bacteria. It is an important mediator of acute inflammation and recruits neutrophils and macrophages to the site of infection by stimulating endothelial cells to produce adhesion molecules and chemotactic chemokines. TNF- α also acts on the hypothalamus to produce fever by producing acute phase proteins [25].

Interleukin 1 (IL-1) is another inflammatory cytokine and produced by activated macrophages. Its effects are similar to that of TNF-α. It also helps to activate T cells [25].

Interleukin 10 (IL-10) is produced by activated macrophages and Th2 cells. Unlike other cytokines, IL-10 functions as an inhibitory cytokine. IL-10 inhibits production of IFN-γ by Th1 cells and also inhibits cytokine production by activated macrophages and the expression of class II MHC and co-stimulatory molecules on macrophages [25].

Interleukin 12 (IL-12) is produced by activated macrophages and dendritic cells and also stimulates the production of IFN-γ. IL-12 also induces the differentiation of Th cells to become Th1 cells. It also enhances the cytolytic functions of cytotoxic T cells and NK cells [25].

Type I interferons especially IFN-α and IFN-β are produced by many cell type and they function to inhibit viral replication in cells. Type I interferon also activates NK cells and increases expression of class I MHC molecules on cells making them more susceptible to killing by CTLs [25].

Interferon gamma (INF-γ) is an important cytokine primarily produced by Th1 cells, and to a lesser extent by Tc and NK cells [25].

Chemokines, also known as chemotactic cytokines are produced by different types leukocytes and other cell types. They represent a large family of molecules and recruit leukocytes to sites of infection and play a role in lymphocyte trafficking [25].

Mediators of Adaptive Immunity

Cytokines belonging to this group are: IL-2, IL-4, IL-5, TGF-β, IL-10 and IFN-γ [25].

Interleukin 2 (IL-2) is primarily produced by Th cells, and to a lesser extent by Tc cells. It is a major growth factor for T cells and also promotes growth of B cells. It also activates NK cells and monocytes. IL-2 acts on T cells in an autocrine manner. Activated T cells express IL-2R and produce IL-2. The IL-2 binds to the IL-R and promotes cell division. When the T cells are no longer stimulated by antigen, the IL-2R decays and proliferation ceases [25].

IL-4 is produced by macrophages and Th2 cells. It stimulates the development of Th2 cells from naive Th cells and promotes its differentiation into Th2 cells for antibody response. It also stimulates Ig class switching to the IgE isotype [25].

IL-5 is produced by Th2 cells. It promotes the growth and differentiation of B cells and eosinophiles. It also activates mature eosinophiles [25].

TGF-β (transforming growth factor beta) is produced by T cells and many other cell types. It is an inhibitory cytokine. TGF- β inhibits the proliferation of T cells and the activation of macrophages. It also acts on PMNs and endothelial cells to block the effects of pro-inflammatory cytokines [25].

Stimulators of Haematopoiesis

A number of cytokines stimulate the differentiation of hematopoetic cells. These include granulocyte macrophage colony stimulating factor (GM-CSF) which stimulates the differentiation of bone-marrow progenitors, macrophage stimulating factor (M-CSF) which promotes growth and differentiation of progenitors into monocytes and macrophages and granulocyte colony stimulating factor (G-CSF) which promotes production of PMNs [25].

Cytokines Involved in Antitumor Response

Interferons

Growing tumor cells release inflammatory cytokines. These cytokines recruit more immune cells which produce pro-inflammatory cytokines such as IL-12, IFN-γ, type I interferons ((IFN-δ/β) *etc.* Of these, IFN-γ and (IFN-δ/β) mediate critical but distinct functions in tumor immunosurveillance [25, 26].

IFN-γ is known to play key role in tumor suppression. NK, NKT and γδ T cells are the major sources of IFN-γ at the early stages of tumor development. CD4+ and CD8+ T cells are thought to become additional sources of IFN-γ as adaptive immunity evolves. IFN-γ contributes to tumor protection in multiple: inhibition of angiogenesis, induction of phagocyte cytotoxicity and stimulation of dendritic cells to produce IL-12 which in turn promotes Th1 and cytotoxic T-cell responses [25, 26].

IFN-γ also functions as a master regulator of tumor cell immunogenicity. More recently IFN-γ has been implicated in the promotion of carcinogenesis. The proposed mechanism showed the involvement of chemokines from damaged skin which attracts IFN-γ secreting macrophages that in turn activate melanocytes [25, 26].

In addition to IFN-γ, type I interferons (IFN-δ/β) in tumor suppression have been defined too. Protection in these systems showed the involvement of host immunity and p53 tumor suppressor function in cancer cells. Clinically, exogenous IFN-α interferon administration showed beneficial effect in hematologic malignancies and melanoma [25, 26].

IL-12 and IL-18

IL-12 and IL-18 are secreted by phagocytic cells, which in turn stimulate innate and adaptive cells to produce IFN-gamma and leads to tumor suppression. Of these, IL-12 enhances NK and NKT cells antitumor activities through NKG2D and perforin dependent pathways. On the other hand, IL-18 augments NK cell cytotoxicity in a NKG2D independent manner that involves Fas ligand mediated apoptotic killing [25, 26].

IL-23 and IL-17

IL-23 is secreted by activated macrophages and dendritic cells. In fact IL-23 and IL-12 share a unique p19 subunit and both IL-12 and IL-23 trigger distinct downstream effector pathways. Whereas IL-12 promotes the development of IFN-gamma secreting Th1 cells, IL-23 supports the expansion and activation of Th17 cells. IL-23 stimulates increased expression of IL-17 which may promote tumor cell growth and invasion through the up-regulation of MMP9, COX-2 and angiogenesis [25, 26].

TH17 cells and IL-17 played some role in promoting IFN-gamma+ effector T cells and NK cells in the tumor microenvironment and showed enhanced tumor immunity. However, IL-17 was shown to be involved in tumor progression in some cases [25, 26].

GM-CSF

Granulocyte-macrophage colony-stimulating factor (GM-CSF) stimulates the production, proliferation, maturation and activation of granulocytes, macrophages and dendritic cells and plays critical role in immune homeostasis. This in turn promotes phagocytosis of apoptotic tumor cells to facilitate antigen presentation to effector lymphocytes with the induction of regulatory T cells and myeloid suppressor cells. GM-CSF has been used as immune adjuvant for cancer vaccines [25, 26].

Antitumor Effector Mechanism Involving Cytotoxic Mechanisms

These include perforin and TNF family members.

Perforin

Cytotoxicity triggered by perforin-granzyme pathways is critical to tumor suppression [1].

TNF

Death receptors belonging to the tumor necrosis factor (TNF) superfamily constitute the second major mechanism of cellular cytotoxicity. TNF-related apoptotsis-inducing ligand (TRAIL) is a type II membrane protein that binds to five receptors in humans. Among these receptors, DR4 (TRAIL-R1) and DR5 (TRAIL-R2) transduce death signals through caspase-8, FADD and Bax. The remaining receptors which are TRAIL-R3, TRAIL-R4 and osteoprotegrin, may attenuate killing as non-signalling receptor decoys. TRAIL is upregulated in various innate and adaptive lymphocytes through interferons (IL-2 and IL-15). The IFN-γ dependent induction of TRAIL on NK cells is critical for the antitumor effects of IL-12 and alpha-GalCer. TRAIL deficiency augments the development of liver metastasis. The therapeutic potential of recombinant TRAIL or anti-TRAIL receptor antibodies in combination with chemotherapy is being tested in humans [1].

Interaction of Fas and Fas ligand triggers anti-tumor cytotoxicity and contribute to control metastasis [1].

LIGHT, another TNF member in tumor suppression functions as a co-stimulatory molecule and triggers an anti-tumor T cell response that mediates destruction of established tumors [25].

Links Between Adaptive and Innate Immunity

A number of cells of the innate immunity play important roles in establishing link between the innate immunity and the adaptive immunity. These are the dendritic cells (DCs) and macrophages. Almost every cell in our body expresses cell surface molecule encoded by genes in the major histocompatibility complex (MHC). MHC class I molecules are found on all nucleated cells excluding the red blood cells as these cells do not have any nucleus and class II molecules are found only on antigen presenting cells such as dendritic cells, macrophages, B cells, thymic epithelial cells *etc.* Cytotoxic T cells recognize peptides on class I MHC molecules and helper T cells recognize class II MHC molecules [1].

Cancer cells also induce inflammatory response. The inflammatory response is a complex process and occurs in four general consecutive phases: (i) pathogen recognition, (ii) recruitment of immune cells to the site of infection, (iii) pathogen elimination and (iv) resolution of inflammation. This sequence of events is initiated by resident macrophages or dendritic cells (DCs) and sometimes by a subset of resident monocytes. The later ones patrol the luminal endothelial surface in healthy tissues and can rapidly invade damaged or infected sites and differentiate into macrophages. Dyeing necrotic cells release damage/pathogen-associated molecular patterns (DAMP/PAMP). These are recognized by the pattern recognition receptors (PRR) expressed by the macrophages and DCs leading to their activation and secretion of pro-inflammatory cytokines. The initial role of macrophage activation is to condition the vasculature of affected tissues for leukocyte infiltration. This process is mediated by factors that induce vasodilation (*e.g.*, histamine, prostaglandins, nitric oxide) and vascular permeability (*e.g.*, histamine, leukotrienes) and the expression of leukocyte adhesion molecules on endothelial cells. Macrophages secrete the cytokines IL-1, IL-8 and tumor necrosis factor-α (TNF- α) as adhesion molecules. These also function to enhance the immune response by triggering a cascade of cells that collectively fight against the infection [1].

Activated macrophages (MQs) and monocytes sense the tissue damage signals such as reactive oxygen species or necrosis associated proteins and other DAMPs. Once activated, MQs induce the production of neutrophil-attracting chemokines and matrix metalloproteinases (MMP) through the neutrophil chemokine receptor CXCR2. Activated neutrophils are forced across post-capillary venules and enter the interstitial space, releasing secretory vesicles containing proteins such as azurocidin and CAP18 *etc.* which activate the endothelial cells and increase vessel permeability. The neutrophils discharge granular cargo of antimicrobial proteins and proteases to further increase the recruitment of inflammatory monocytes by various mechanisms. These monocytes with recruited neutrophils and macrophages eliminate the damage-inflicting source. Finally, a switch in lipid signalling from pro-inflammatory prostaglandins and leukotrienes to anti-inflammatory prostaglandins and lipoxins block further recruitment of neutrophils and induce their apoptosis and clearance by macrophages. This enables the resolution of inflammation and the reestablishment of tissue homeostasis [3, 15, 27].

DC and macrophages possess pathogen recognition receptor (PRR) that detect pathogen-associated molecular patterns (PAMPs) on the microbes. PRRs are of several types such as secreted, cytosolic and transmembrane classes. Of these, Toll-like receptors or TLR, are present on the plasma membrane and NOD-like receptors are present in the cytosol [3, 15, 27].

Unlike macrophages, DCs destroy pathogens by communicating with the adaptive immune system and thereby confer long lasting antigen-specific immune responses [3, 15, 27]. DCs accomplish this function by collecting the proteolytic apparatus in both the endosomal-lysosomal system (mediated by cathepsins and other lysosomal hydrolases) as well as in the cytosol (proteasome) and endoplasmic reticulum (ER). In fact DCs are capable of capturing even very small amounts of antigen for presentation. These help to partially degrade pathogen derived proteins to yield antigenic peptides that in turn are loaded onto MHC class I or class II molecules. More specifically, MHC class I is associated with the presentation of peptides derived from antigens synthesized endogenously. Example of this class is viral antigens. On the other hand, MHC class II presents antigens derived from extracellular sources. These antigens are from bacteria, protozoa, allergens or dead cells that are internalized by endocytosis and delivered to one or more populations of endosomes and lysosomes where the invaders encounter acidic environments [3, 15, 27].

In immature DCs, MHC class II molecules are delivered to the same compartments and the denatured and partially cleaved antigen domains bind to the MHC class II binding cleft. The unbound regions of the protein are removed by exo-proteases whereas 10-15 mer peptide remains bound with the MHC class II binding cleft. Upon maturation, the peptide-MHC complexes are transferred to the surface of the DC cells or are routed there constitutively if formed after maturation [3, 15, 27].

The resulting peptide-MHC complexes are transported to the plasma membrane where they are presented to their cognate T cells leading to the activation and induction of the T cells to proliferate into potent effector cells (cytotxic T cells) or helper T cells. DCs also express ligands, *e.g.*, CD80 and CD86 that bind to costimulatory molecules on T cells that act in concert with the peptide-MHC specific T-cell receptor. DCs also produce stimulatory cytokines, *e.g.*, interleukin 12 (IL-12) that are required for optimal stimulation of T cells. DCs also can stimulate B cells directly by presenting intact antigen at the DCs surface, thereby activating B cells cognate specificity [3, 15, 27].

Toll-like Receptor (TLR) Signalling

TLRs are a family of transmembrane protein that recognize conserved molecular patterns of microbial origin. TLRs play crucial role upon tissue damage by regulating tissue repair and inflammation. Ligands of TLRs can be exogenous (*e.g.* microbial pathogen associated molecular patterns (PAMPs) or endogenous (*e.g.*, heat-shock protein/HSP and uric acid crystals). Different ligands are recognized by different TLRs. For example, lipopolysaccharide is recognized by TLR-4, and bacterial flagellin by TLR-5. Different TLRs are localized in different subcellular compartments. For *e.g.*, TLRs that recognize lipid or protein ligands are expressed on the plasma membrane (TLR-1,-2, -4, -5, -6) and TLRs that respond to viral nucleic acids are in the endolysosomal compartment (TLR-3, -7, -9). Upon binding of the ligand, one or more adapter proteins (*e.g.*, MyD88 and TICAM1) transmit the intracellular signal [3, 28].

TLRs play important role in host defense against infections, tissue repair and regeneration and even in cancer. Polymorphisms in TLRs are associated with human breast, stomach and colon cancers. TLRs have both negative and positive regulatory properties during tumorogenesis. Anticancer effect of TLRs was observed both in human and mice after injecting purified TLR ligands which increased apoptosis of tumor cells, recruitment of NK and cytotoxic T cells and stimulation of adaptive immune response, thereby breaking tolerance to tumor self-antigens. TLRs are also important for the recognition of viral pathogens that can promote development of cancer (*e.g.* Epstein–Barr virus, hepatitis B and C viruses, human papillomavirus, and *Helicobacter pylori*). TLR signalling has also been reported to promote the growth and survival of tumor cells involving MyD88 signalling during the development of colitis and colitis-associated colon cancer in murine models. These pleiotropic functions of TLR signalling during tissue repair and tumorigenesis is thought to be dependent on the respective milieu, cell type and type of TLR signalling [3, 28].

Inflammasomes

The inflammasomes are a large protein complex with the capacity to sense various PAMP and DAMP. Inflammasomes are expressed in DCs, macrophages and epithelial cells. Upon activation, inflammasomes initiate immune response toward the invading pathogen or tissue damage by the sensory components of the inflammasome which is known as NOD-like receptors (NLR). NODs constitute a large family of cytosolic PRRs and composed of a C-terminal leucine rich repeat domain (LRR), a central neucleotide-binding domain (NBD) and an N-terminal pyrin domain (PYD). Of these three domains, LRR and NBD modules are thought to be involved in ligand sensing and PYD is involved in the recruitment of adapter protein ASC (apoptosis associated speck-like protein containing a caspase-associated and recruitment domain (CARD)). ASC is associated with pro-caspas--1. The ternary protein complex formed by NLRs, ASC and caspase-1 is known as inflammasome [3].

Activation of inflammasome complex leads to auto-cleavage and activation of pro-caspase-1 which in turn secrete proinflammatory cytokines IL-1β and IL-18 and IL-33 and FGF-2. The activation of inflammasome leads to pyroptosis. Unlike classical apoptosis, pyroptosis promotes local inflammation associated with the release of IL-1β and IL-18, and this mechanism of cell death is important to promote both the suicide of engulfed macrophages and cell-autonomous tumor suppression. Overall, inflammasomes play critical role in tumor growth by sensing the environment and modulating two key aspects of inflammation: proinflammatory cytokine activation and cell death [3].

Specific Interplay of Innate and Adaptive Antitumor Immunity

Innate immunity stimulates the generation of adaptive immune response through the presentation of tumor antigens by dendritic cells. The detection of danger signals elicited by stress or cell death and interactions with other innate cells trigger dendritic cell activation. In this way, NK cells that recognize NKG2D ligand-positive, MHC class I-deficient tumors, NKT cells that detect CD1d presented lipids, and γδ T cells that recognize stress antigens interact productively with dendritic cells. In this cross talk, cytokines (mentioned above), B7 family members, and CD40 play critical roles [1, 29].

Another example of the involvement of DCs in antitumor response can be cited by the MUC1 antigen processing. MUC1 antigen is categorized as over-expressed tumor antigen. Immune responses to MUC1 in both normal and healthy individuals have been studied in terms of the normal and tumor form of MUC1 for its ability to be processed and presented by dendritic cells and activate helper T cells. Fully glycosylated form of MUC1 can be uptaken by DC but it is not trafficked into antigen-processing compartments and not cleaved into antigenic peptides. On the other hand, tumor form that lacks sugars completely or is only sparsely glycosylated with short sugars leaving large stretches of the polypeptide core unprotected, can be processed into peptides and glycopeptides, both presented on the DC surface in MHC class II molecules. Both peptide specific and glycopeptides specific T cells were primed with these DCs [22].

IMMUNE-ESCAPE

Despite that our immune system shows antitumor response, there are ample evidence that shows that tumors do develop even in the presence of an active and efficient immune response. This process is known as immuno-escape and several mechanism are involved with the process [7, 29].

Signalling Defects in Anti-tumor T Cells

Research on signalling defects in T cells are now-a days broadly emphasized on the development of T cells that are unable to perform effector functions intrinsic to their type of functional differentiation, and also to the development of T cells that have differentiated toward the erroneous functional programs instead of suppressing the tumor progression.

Functional differentiation, also termed 'polarization' of T cells is regulated by several types of signals present in the environment at the time of initial antigen recognition and activation. The different functional programs include: T helper (Th) 1, Th2, Th17, and regulatory T-cells (Treg) differentiation. Multiple factors including the strength of T-cell receptor (TCR) mediated signals and cytokines play important role to influence naïve $CD4^+$ T cell differentiation. Th1 differentiation is initiated by IFN-γ which is produced by NK cells, CD8+ or other CD4+ T cells and is sustained by IL-12. On the other hand Th2 differentiation is driven by IL-4 (*e.g.* produced by basophils) and Th2 transcription factor GATA-3 suppresses expression of the TH1 transcription factor T-bet. Th17 differentiation is dependent on the presence of transforming growth factor β (TGF-β) and IL-6 and their differentiation is mutually exclusive with adaptive or induced Treg (iTreg) differentiation which requires TGF-β and IL-2 [7, 29].

The lack of tumor antigen (TA) recognition has been attributed to the loss of signal transducers chain (CD3-γ) of TILs to immune evasion in the co-operation of immunosuppressive cytokines and local impairment CD3-γ of TILs. The loss of CD3-γ is correlated with increased levels of IL-10 and TGF-β and down-regulation of IFN-γ. The CD3-γ chain is located as a large inracytoplasmic homodimer in the TCR and forms TCR-CD3 complex. This functions as a single transducer upon antigen binding. TCR signal transduction through the formation of CD3 complex is one of the three important signals for initiating a successful immune response. Any alteration in this CD3-γ chain is associated with the absence of p56lck tyrosine kinase, but not CD3-Ɛ, producing changes in the signalling pathway for T-cell activation. The alterations of TCR-γ have been associated with poor prognosis in several types of tumors such as pancreatic cancer, uveal malignant melanoma, renal cell cancer, ovarian cancer and oral cancer. Defective TCR-γ expression leads to poor proliferative response of TILs. Research showed that TIL underwent marked spontaneous apoptosis *in vitro* which was associated with down-regulation of the anti-apoptotic Bcl-xL and Bcl-2 proteins. Furthermore, TCR-γ is a substrate of caspase 3 leading to apoptosis. Tumor cells can trigger caspase-dependent apoptotic cascades in T lymphocytes, and are not protected by Bcl-2. It was also reported that in oral squamous cell carcinoma, significant proportion of T cells undergo apoptosis which is correlated with high FasL expression on tumor cells. FasL positive microvesicles induced caspase-3 cleavage which eventually triggered cytochrome-c release, loss of mitochondrial membrane potential and reduced TCR-γ chain expression in target lymphocytes [7, 29].

Tumor Derived Factors

A variety of tumor derived soluble factors contribute to the emergence of complex local and regional immunosuppressive networks that can lead to malignant progression. These include vascular endothelial growth factor (VEGF), IL-10, TGF-b, prostaglandin E_2, soluble phosphatidylserine, soluble Fas, soluble FasL and soluble MICA. Although these soluble factors are deposited at the primary tumor site, these can extend immunosuppressive effects into local lymph nodes and the spleen to promote invasion and metastasis [20].

VEGF plays a key role in recruiting immature myeloid cells from the bone marrow to enrich the microenvironment with tumor-associated immature DCs (TiDCs) and macrophages (TAM). Accumulation of TiDCs can cause the moving DCs and T cells to become suppressed through activation of indoleamine 2,3-dioxygenase (IDO) and arginase I by tumor-derived growth factors. VEGF prevents DC differentiation and maturation by suppressing the nuclear factor- κB in haematopoietic stem cells. Also, VEGF can be activated by signal transducers and activators of transcription factors 3 (STAT3). Since DC differentiation requires decreasing activity of Stat3, neutralizing VEGF or Sta3 activation can promote DC differentiation and function. The increased serum levels of VEGF in cancers have been reported to be correlated with poor prognosis involving its angiogenic properties and induction of immune evasion leading to tumor progression [20].

Soluble FasL and MICA inhibit Fas-mediated and NKG2D-mediated killing of immune cells and thereby play important roles in immune evasion. Soluble phosphatidylserine (PS) acts as an inducer of anti-inflammatory mediators such as IL-10 and TGF-β that inhibit immune responses of DCs and T cells [1].

Chemokines in Promoting Cancer Development

Cancer cells express an extensive network of chemokines and chemokine receptors. These chemokines are chemo-attractant and induced by cytokines, growth factors and pathogenic stimuli. The molecular weight of these proteins ranges from 8-10 kDa. The chemokines are divided into four groups, C, CC, CXC and CX3C. The grouping is based on the number and the spacing of the first two cysteine residues in the amino-terminal part of the protein. Chemokines orchestrate cell movement during homeostatic trafficking of haematopoietic stem cells, lymphocytes and dendritic cells and also during any inflammatory response. Chemokines exert their effect by binding to the extracellular N-terminus of the chemokine receptors which are the seven-transmembrane domain G protein-coupled receptors (7TM-GPCR). Once bind to the receptor, this leads to phosphporylation of serine/threonine residues on the cytoplasmic C-terminus, signalling and then receptor desensitisation. Once the chemokine binds to its receptors, it stimulates transcription of genes involved in invasion, motility, extracellular matrix interaction and cell survival [26]. Chemokines have both pro-apoptotic function and anti-cancer action. Table **3** shows some of the chemokine receptors expressed by different cancer cells (Table **3**).

Table 3. Tumor and stroma derived chemokines [21, 26].

Ligand	Producing tumors
CXC family	
CXCL1/Groa	Colon carcinoma
CXCL8/IL-8	Melanoma
CXCL9/Mig	Hodgkin's disease
CXCL10/IP-10	Hodgkin's lymphoma and nasopharyngeal carcinoma
CXCL13/BCA1	Non-Hodgkin's B cell lymphoma
CXCR3	Melanoma

(Table 3) contd.....

Ligand	Producing tumors
CXCR4	Breast, colorectal, esophageal, glioma, melanoma, nasopharangeal, non-small-cell lung, osteosarcoma, obarian, pancreatic, prostate, renal and thyroid cancer.
CXCR5	Head and neck
CC family	
CCL1/I-309	Adult T cell leukemia
CCL2/MCP-1	Pancreas, sarcomas, gliomas, lung, breast, cervix, ovary, melanoma
CCL3/MIP-1a	Schwann cell tumors
CCL3L1/LD78b	Glioblastoma
CCL5/RANTES	Breast
CCL6	Non-small-cell lung
CCL7/MCP-3	Osteosarcoma
CCL8/MCP-3	Osteosarcoma
CCL11/eotaxin	T-cell lymphoma
CCL17/TARC	Lymphoma
CCL18/PARC	Ovary
CCL22/MDC	Ovary
CCL28/MEC	Hodgkin's disease
CCR3	Renal
CCR4	ATLL
CCR5	Prostate
CCR7	Breast, colorectal, esophageal, gastric, non-small cell lung, oral/oropharangeal
CCR9	Melanoma
CCR10	Melanoma
CX3 family	
CX3CR1	Prostate

Tumor-associated chemokines play several roles in the biology of primary and metastatic diseases. These are: control of leukocyte infiltration into the tumor, manipulation of tumor immune response, regulation of angiogenesis, action as autocrine or paracrine growth and survival factors, and direct the movement of the tumor cells themselves [26].

Tumor Associated Myeloid Derived Suppressor Cells

Myeloid derived suppressor cells (MDSC) are a population of early myeloid cells that originate from bone marrow stem cells and are expanded at various disease states including cancer. Although these cells also include the dendritic cells, macrophages and neutrophils, MDSC are capable of suppressing the immune response instead of antitumor response [31].

MDSC are a heterogenous population of precursor myeloid cells that are known to cause immune suppression. In healthy population, MDSC is low as myeloid progenitors differentiate normally into mature myeloid cells. However, under pathological conditions, maturation is arrested at various stages and the cells take on a suppressive capacity. Tumor-derived proinflammatory cytokines IL-6 and IL-1β, promote the formation of MDSCs which leads to the accumulation of these cells in the bloods, lymphoid organs and tumor. In cancer the ratio of mature DCs to immature myeloid cells in the blood is inversely proportional to the stage of the disease. The expression markers for MDSC are different in human and mice. For example, in humans, MDSC cells are identified by the expression marker CD33, CD11b and IL-4Rα. In mice, CD11b and GR1 are universally expressed and there is no human homolog for this. Other cytokines and growth factors such as GM-CSF, G-CSF, IL-10, vascular endothelial growth factor (VEGF), prostaglandin E2 (PGE-2) and IL-1 have been implicated in the development and regulation of MDSC [31].

MDSCs are further divided into two groups. The grouping is based on nuclear morphology. These are: the granulocytic MDSC and the monocytic MDSC. The former ones are polymorphonuclear and the later ones are mononuclear. MDSCs also express other surface markers such as ICAM-1, CD80 and CD15, and exhibit great variability between individuals depending on the type of tumor [31].

MDSCs exhibit diverse immune suppression effects and this happens either directly or indirectly. MDSCs directly inhibit CD8+ and CD4+ T cells in a cell contact dependent manner through arginine and systeine depletion. Both the amino acids are essential for T cell activation. MDSCs also can inhibit T cell function through the production of reactive oxygen species (ROS). Monocytic MDSCs elevate iNOS, which suppresses antigen-specific T cells by increasing nitrosylation of MHC. MDSC also inhibit through antigen-independent mechanisms. They reduce the expression of L-selectin on naïve T cells which prevent their circulation through lymph nodes and tumors, eventually leading to reduced number of active T cells. Another indirect mechanism by which MDSCs suppress immune system is by inducing Tregs. Treg induction occurs through CD40 expression on MDSCs [31].

Antigen Specific T-cell Tolerance

Many tumor cells are capable of inducing protective cyto-toxic T-cell response which was evidenced by transferring a single-cell cell suspension. However, if these are transplanted as small tumor pieces (size approximately of 1 mm^3) in SCID mice, the tumors readily grow because the tumor antigen level can be modulated in the tumor micro-environment. These can be explained by the fact that tumor cells are surrounded by non-tumor cells, including bone-marrow derived cells such as iDCs and non-bone-marrow-derived cells such as fibroblasts, endothelium and ECM. The ECM binds with the tumor antigens and fibroblasts and endothelial cells compete with DCs for the antigen. This results in the down-regulation of many tumor antigen, allowing tumor progression. These stromal cells also increase interstitial fluid pressure in the tumor, resulting in escape from immune attacks by effector cells. iDCs not only suppress T-cell function, they also stimulate CD4$^+$CD25$^+$ regulatory T cells, which inhibit T-cell activation. Even in the presence of sufficient tumor antigens, iDCs inhibit the maturation of DCs and T-cell activation, resulting in immunological tolerance, which results in tumor immune evasion which is mediated by immunological ignorance and also by immunological tolerance because of inhibition of T-cell activation by iDCs [10].

Regulatory T (Treg) Cells

Tumor cells escape immune detection by avoiding self-recognition. Regulatory immune cells are a diverse group of cells of the adaptive and innate immune cell subsets that prevent autoimmunity by suppressing self recognizing T cells. Tumor cells secrete certain types of cytokines into the tumor microenvironment. These promote differentiation of many types of regulatory cells that reduces the activity of effector T cells targeted toward the tumor. The two main types of regulatory cells are CD4+CD25hiFoxP3+T cells (Tregs) and myeloid derived suppressor cells (MDSCs) [7, 31].

Many tumor cells produce TGF-β, which promotes differentiation of naïve CD4+ T cells into Tregs. Increased Treg frequency is correlated with poor outcome. In animal models, selective depletion of Tregs enhanced tumor regression. Tregs inhibit antigen presenting cells (APCs) by inducing upregulation of inhibitory B7-H4 molecules or by direct killing releasing perforin and granzymes. Tregs engage CD80/86 on APCs with cytotoxic T lymphocyte antigen 4 (CTLA-4), leading to T cell anergy and death. Finally, these regulatory cells secrete immunosuppressive cytokines such as IL-10 and TGF-β to preserve and spread immunosuppression within the tumor microenvironment [7, 31].

IMMUNE-EVASION

Immuno-evasion is the other mechanism adopted by tumor cells to avoid immune detection. For example, tumors down-regulate expression of MHC class I and other proteins that are involved in antigen presentation. Tumors can also decrease or shed expression of proteins that are recognized by the immuno system. In addition, tumors can by-pass death mechanisms by elevating expression levels of cell survival proteins such as anti-apopottic proteins (*e.g.*, surviving, BCL-XL), metastatic proteins (VEGF, MMPs), and proliferation factors (EGFR, c-Myc). In addition, certain transcription factors (discussed in chapter 3) (*e.g.*, STAT3, p53 *etc.*) are upregulated in several tumors which further controls the upregulation of some of the oncogenes. Also the tumor microenvironment is populated with heterogenous cell types which are at various states of development. As a result, it helps the tumor cells to evolve quickly in response to new stresses. Tumor cells adapt to immuno recognition by down regulating the expression of antigens, or can adapt to chemotherapy drugs by increasing expression of metabolic pathway associated proteins or by increasing expression of adenosine-triphosphate binding cassette (ABC) pumps to actively secrete intracellular drugs. However, a successful chemotherapy regiment can also increase the chance of recurrence as there are few resistant cells that survive the treatment and can seed a secondary malignancy [29].

Circulating Tumor Cells

Circulating tumor cells (CTC) are those tumor cells that actively leave tumor, survive in circulation and then actively invade into distant organs where they proliferate and form new tumors. CTC are associated with distant metastasis in cancers like colorectal cancer and are associated with poor prognosis (reference: Circulating tumor cells of colorectal cancer). CTC develops a certain phenotype (metastatic) which is accomplished by multistep processes: bulk tumor cells initially undergo epithelial-mesenchymal transition (EMT) to acquire a mesenchymal phenotype to invade the blood vessels. Once they enter the blood stream (also known as intravasation), the tumor cells shift to an immune-evasive state (IES) to be able to cloak from immune cells. The tumor cells then enter the epithelium of the target organs and acquire an invasive phenotype to enter the target organ (also called extravasation). Afterwards, the cells undergo MET and proliferate as epithelial tumor cells. Since CTC cells need to switch from EMT (epithelial-mesenchymal transition) to mesenchymal-epithelial transition (MET) during which invasion of target organs such as the liver shows phenotypically quite similar to the primary tumor, it is a question of long debate why the immune system fails to recognize and clear all putative circulating tumor cells from the blood stream. Research on this showed that CTC cells express CD47 markers, which is a "don't-eat-me" signal and prevents immune cells such as the NK cells, monocytes/macrophages from killing CTC. Up-regulation of CD47 exhibited down-regulation of other genes such as Ki-67 and c-Myc which are associated with cell death mechanism. On the other hand, calreticulin (CALR), a "chaperon" protein expressed on damaged cells stimulates immune cells to kill the damaged cells that are significantly down regulated on CTC [30, 32].

The ultimate goal of CTC phenotyping efforts is to identify a therapeutic target to prevent the occurrence of distant metastasis and tumor recurrence in early stage patients [32].

CONCLUSION

An effective immune response is characterized by specificity, trafficking, adaptability and durability or memory. Specificity ensures that an immune response is targeted toward specific antigens; trafficking refers to the ability of activated immune cells to migrate to particular antigens throughout the body. Adaptability is the third characteristic of an effective immune response is target adaptability. It allows expansion of the immune response beyond the initially targeted antigen through a process known as epitope and antigen spreading. Epitope spreading occurs when immune cells are able to generate an immune response to other epitopes or region of the target antigens. On the other hand, antigen spreading occurs when immune cells are able to generate an immune response to related antigens originating from the same cell. Finally, durability or memory refers to the ability of T cells to recognize antigen over time. Immunologic memory allows for an expedited and durable immune response upon re-exposure to antigens. At present, inflammation, immune evasion and immune-escape mechanisms are considered as hallmarks of cancer cells. Cancer cells are gradually able to gain immune evasion during tumor progression. In advanced cancers, the marked shifting to immune-suppressive conditions, make it difficult to induce an active immune response. Therefore, to design an effective immunotherapy drug, it needs to be ensured that the drug contains the essential characteristics of the effective immune system. Also, extensive information on the tumor microenvironment and cell signalling molecules are required to understand the molecular and cellular level of the cell under perturbed conditions.

CONFLICT OF INTEREST

The author confirms that author has no conflict of interest to declare for this publication.

ACKNOWLEDGEMENTS

Declared none.

REFERENCES

[1]   Ploegh HL. Logic of the immune system. Cancer Immunol Res 2013; 1(1): 5-10.
       [http://dx.doi.org/10.1158/2326-6066.CIR-13-0023] [PMID: 24777244]

[2]   Siegel R, Naishadham D, Jemal A. Cancer statistics, 2013. CA Cancer J Clin 2013; 63(1): 11-30.
       [http://dx.doi.org/10.3322/caac.21166] [PMID: 23335087]

[3]   Nowarski R, Gagliani N, Huber S, Flavell RA. Innate immune cells in inflammation and cancer.

Cancer Immunol Res 2013; 1(2): 77-84.
[http://dx.doi.org/10.1158/2326-6066.CIR-13-0081] [PMID: 24777498]

[4]   Robins R. Cancer Immunology. Book 2001; 1-3.

[5]   Grivennikov SI, Greten FR, Karin M. Immunity, inflammation, and cancer. Cell 2010; 140(6): 883-99.
        [http://dx.doi.org/10.1016/j.cell.2010.01.025] [PMID: 20303878]

[6]   Mian S, Robins RA, Rees RC, Fox B. Cancer Immunology 2014; 1-6.

[7]   Dudek AM, Martin S, Garg AD, Agostinis P. Immature, semi-mature, and fully mature dendritic cells:
        toward a DC-cancer cells interface that augments anticancer immunity. Front Immunol 2013; 4: 438.
        [http://dx.doi.org/10.3389/fimmu.2013.00438] [PMID: 24376443]

[8]   Flavell RA, Mellman I. Cancer Immunology Essentials Logic of the Immune System Cancer
        Immunology Essentials. 2014; 1-2.

[9]   Peng G. Characterization of regulatory T cells in tumor suppressive microenvironments. Methods Mol
        Biol 2010; 651: 31-48.
        [http://dx.doi.org/10.1007/978-1-60761-786-0_2] [PMID: 20686958]

[10]   Kim R, Emi M, Tanabe K. Cancer immunoediting from immune surveillance to immune escape.
        Immunology 2007; 121(1): 1-14.
        [http://dx.doi.org/10.1111/j.1365-2567.2007.02587.x] [PMID: 17386080]

[11]   Bessoles S, Grandclément C, Alari-Pahissa E, Gehrig J, Jeevan-Raj B, Held W. Adaptations of natural
        killer cells to self-MHC class I. Front Immunol 2014; 5: 349.
        [http://dx.doi.org/10.3389/fimmu.2014.00349] [PMID: 25101089]

[12]   Lin H, Gordon S. Macrophage phenotype in tumor. In: Lawrence T, Hagemann T, Eds. Tumor assoc
        macrophages springer science+ business media. LLC Landes Bioscience 2012; pp. 3-16.

[13]   Noy R, Pollard JW. Tumor-associated macrophages: from mechanisms to therapy. Immunity 2014;
        41(1): 49-61.
        [http://dx.doi.org/10.1016/j.immuni.2014.06.010] [PMID: 25035953]

[14]   Mantovani A, Sica A. Macrophages, innate immunity and cancer: balance, tolerance, and diversity.
        Curr Opin Immunol 2010; 22(2): 231-7.
        [http://dx.doi.org/10.1016/j.coi.2010.01.009] [PMID: 20144856]

[15]   Mellman I. Dendritic cells· master regulators of the immune response. Cancer Immunol Res 2013;
        1(3): 145-9.
        [http://dx.doi.org/10.1158/2326-6066.CIR-13-0102] [PMID: 24777676]

[16]   Gardy JL, Lynn DJ, Brinkman FS, Hancock RE. Enabling a systems biology approach to immunology:
        focus on innate immunity. Trends Immunol 2009; 30(6): 249-62.
        [http://dx.doi.org/10.1016/j.it.2009.03.009] [PMID: 19428301]

[17]   Wilke CM, Wei S, Wang L, *et al.* T cell and antigen-presenting cell subsets in the tumor
        microenvironment. In: Curiel TJ, Ed. Cancer Immunother Springer New York, New York. NY 2013;
        pp. 17-44.
        [http://dx.doi.org/10.1007/978-1-4614-4732-0_2]

[18]   Gajewski TF. Cancer immunotherapy. Mol Oncol 2012; 6(2): 242-50.

[http://dx.doi.org/10.1016/j.molonc.2012.01.002] [PMID: 22248437]

[19]   Chosdol K, Bhagat M, Dikshit B, *et al.* Nuclear factors linking cancer and infl ammation. In: Kumar R, Ed. Nucl signal pathways target transcr cancer springer science+ business media. New York: LLC Landes Bioscience 2014; pp. 121-54.
[http://dx.doi.org/10.1007/978-1-4614-8039-6_6]

[20]   Zhang B, Rowley DA, Schreiber H. Tumor stroma and the antitumor immune response. In: Gabrilovich D, Hurwitz A, Eds. Tumor induc immunesuppression. New York: Springer 2008; pp. 281-94.
[http://dx.doi.org/10.1007/978-0-387-69118-3_13]

[21]   Paschen A, Finn OJ, Binder RJ, *et al.* Tumor-Associated Antigens. 2009. Seliger Copyright

[22]   Finn OJ. Human Tumor Antigens, and Cancer Vaccines. Immunol Res 2006; 73-82.
[http://dx.doi.org/10.1385/IR:36:1:73] [PMID: 17337768]

[23]   Gabrilovich DI, Hurwitz AA, Eds. Tumor Induced Immune Suppression : Mechanisms and Therapeutic Reversal. New York, NY, USA: Springer 2014.

[24]   Vigneron N, Stroobant V, Eynde BJ, Van Den , Bruggen P, Van Der . Database of T cell-defined human tumor antigens. 2013; 13: pp. 1-6.

[25]   Jiang J, Wu C, Lu B. Cytokine-induced killer cells promote antitumor immunity. J Transl Med 2013; 11: 83.
[http://dx.doi.org/10.1186/1479-5876-11-83] [PMID: 23536996]

[26]   Slettenaar VI, Wilson JL. The chemokine network: a target in cancer biology? Adv Drug Deliv Rev 2006; 58(8): 962-74.
[http://dx.doi.org/10.1016/j.addr.2006.03.012] [PMID: 16996642]

[27]   Gabrilovich Dimitry I, Hurwitz Arthur A, Eds. Tumor Induced Immune Suppression : Mechanisms and Therapeutic Reversal. New York, NY, USA: Springer 2014.

[28]   Fukata M, Vamadevan AS, Abreu MT. Toll-like receptors (TLRs) and Nod-like receptors (NLRs) in inflammatory disorders. Semin Immunol 2009; 21(4): 242-53.
[http://dx.doi.org/10.1016/j.smim.2009.06.005] [PMID: 19748439]

[29]   Knutson KL, Disis ML. Tumor antigen-specific T helper cells in cancer immunity and immunotherapy. Cancer Immunol Immunother 2005; 54(8): 721-8.
[http://dx.doi.org/10.1007/s00262-004-0653-2] [PMID: 16010587]

[30]   Steinert G, Schölch S, Niemietz T, *et al.* Immune escape and survival mechanisms in circulating tumor cells of colorectal cancer. Cancer Res 2014; 74(6): 1694-704.
[http://dx.doi.org/10.1158/0008-5472.CAN-13-1885] [PMID: 24599131]

[31]   Serafini P, Bronte V. Myeloid-derived suppressor cells in cancer cells with suppressive activity on the immune response 2008; 157-95.

[32]   Schö S, Bork U, Rahbari NN, Koch M. Circulating tumor cells of colorectal cancer 2014; 1-6.

CHAPTER 2

Cancer Metabolism: A Perspective on the Involvement of the Immune System and Metabolic Pathways in Cancer Development

Abstract: Cancer cells show excessive need of nutrients and energy. Not only this, activated lymphocytes, in particular the T lymphocytes and myeloid derived cells also show differential expression in the metabolic pathway genes in tumor microenvironment. Therefore, understanding the metabolic changes in the context of cancer development will help to identify new therapeutic targets to treat cancer.

Keywords: Arginine metabolism, Autophagy pathway, Immune-metabolism, Immune-suppressors, Leptin, Reactive oxygen species, Tumor metabolism.

INTRODUCTION

The two most fundamental ways in which cells interact with their environment is through metabolism and through immune response. The former one involves obtaining nutrients to sustain life and the later one is to defend against pathogenic organisms. While the former one is generally known as metabolism, the later one is referred to as immune response. For a long time, immunology and metabolism have been addressed as two separate fields of study. However, both processes involve thousands of enzymes, proteins and regulatory molecules which indicate that these processes might be connected and closely interacted to maintain cellular homeostasis. In fact, in the recent years, the field of immune-metabolism has drawn much attention to understand the mechanism by which nutrients affect the immune system in the context of cancer cells. This has emerged as a new field for the development of therapies that can be used as chemotherapy or immunotherapy or a combination therapy [1, 2].

Mahbuba Rahman

Cancer cells show highly complex and dynamic environment in which tumor cells interact with stromal cells within a modified extracellular matrix (ECM). During tumor progression, pervasive stromal cells reprogramme and remodel, and transform a normal environment into tumorogenic microenvironment. Since cancer originates from inflammation, therefore, the tumorigenic micro-environment consists of a variety of mesenchymal immune and inflammatory cells and non-immune stromal cells or fibroblasts. However, fibroblasts, which represent the principal cellular component of tumor microenvironment, become cancer associated fibroblasts (CAF) or myofibroblasts once they are recruited, activated and accumulated to the tumor microenvironment. CAFS are a hetero-geneous cell group originating from various sources. The locally resident stromal cells are considered as a major source of CAFs and they have distinctly different morphological and functional features from their normal counterparts. Bone-marrow derived mesenchymal stem cells (MSCs) serve as another group of CAF. Several studies suggest that tumor epithelial cells induce aerobic glycolysis in neighboring fibroblast. CAFS then secrete lactic acid and pyruvic acid, which are taken up by tumor cells. In fact, the heterotypic interactions between stromal cells and tumor cells with genetic and epigenetic alterations generate numerous adaptive strategies for the tumor cells, giving it a distinct phenotype as compared to the surrounding tissues. The adaptive strategies in tumor microenvironment include plasticity, acquisition of stem-like properties, unfolded protein response, production of exosomes, autophagy, invasion, metabolic reprogramming, immunosuppression and therapeutic resistance. Among these strategies, metabolic and immune reprogramming has been highlighted recently since the immune cells in tumor environment also compete for the nutrient. Therefore, overcoming metabolic stress is a critical step for tumor cells to survive and metastasize [1].

While tumor cells show increased metabolic and energy demand, proliferating T lymphocytes also show similar type of metabolic profiles. Nonetheless, patients with cancer showed impaired T cell response which was found to decrease the potential therapeutic effect of cancer vaccines and other forms of immunotherapy. Therefore, it is important to understand the metabolic profiles of both the tumor cells and T lymphocytes as metabolic reprogramming has been shown to be associated with therapy resistance in cancer cells which is also a part of the immune escape mechanism. In fact, nowadays it is well established that a variety of metabolites (*e.g.*, lactic acid, reactive oxygen species *etc.*) promote tumor progression and also intimate the immune cells for immune escape mechanism. Furthermore, different cytokines (*e.g.*, leptin), secreted by tumor infiltrating immune cells (TILs) also support tumor growth. Apparently, cancer-immune-metabolism is a complex process having potential importance to elucidate the underlying mechanism of therapeutic resistance and development of new drugs or therapies for cancer treatment. Keeping in view the importance of metabolism in supporting cancer development, in this section we will discuss the metabolic reprogramming of cancer cells followed by its importance in assisting tumor cells to adopt the stressful conditions [3, 4].

METABOLIC REPROGRAMMING OF THE IMMUNE CELLS IN TUMOR MICROENVIRONMENT

Interaction of the immune system with tumor complex is a dynamic process as several components of the anti-tumor immunity are involved in eradicating tumor cells. The anti-tumor immune response is mediated by tumor antigen-specific cytotoxic T (CTL) cells and T effector (Teff) cells together with antibody-producing B cells and antigen presenting dendritic cells (DCs). These responses elicit adaptive anti-tumor activity through directly recognizing and removing tumor cells or thorugh cross-talk between the adaptive and innate immune responses. In addition, macrophages, natural killer (NK) cells, and NK-T cells form an important layer of non-specific immunity to suppress tumor progression [5, 6].

A proper immune system must have appropriate and sufficient energy to perform their function in response to non-self-particles or antigens. Accordingly, metabolic regulation and cell signalling are tightly and ubiquitously linked with immune response. The distinct metabolic profiles of different lymphocytes are intimately linked to their status and function. For example, resting cells are quiescent and rely only on adenosine triphosphate (ATP) for basal cell functions. Naïve T lymphocytes rely mainly on fatty acid oxidation and glycolysis to fulfill their energy demand for survival. However, to provide protection against the pathogen, T cells must remain capable of rapid responses and effector function.

This means that a diverse pool of naïve lymphocytes should be quickly activated to produce a large, clonal pool of rapidly proliferating effector T cells [5, 6].

Naïve T cells express T cell antigen receptors (TCR) which are randomly generated through V(D)J recombination and pre-selected to recognize foreign antigens presented on major histocompatibility complexes (MHC). These naïve cells continuously circulate the blood and lymphatic system in search for foreign antigens that are in complex form of MHC-peptide complexes on antigen presenting cells (APCs). Once the T cell encounters the APCs and the cognate antigen, its migration ceases to form prolonged contact with the APCs. This interaction induces signaling through the TCR and other co-receptors and induces T cell activation, proliferation and differentiation into effector T cells [5, 6].

The effector T cells rapidly accumulate and migrate to sites of inflammation to destroy the pathogens. However, upon stimulation, lymphocytes enter the cell cycle and divide within 4-6 hours, a process which requires both energy in the form of ATP and biomolecules for rapid cell growth. During this process, T lymphocytes reprogram their metabolism where glycolysis coupled with glutamine metabolism provides both ATP and synthesis of the biomolecules, such as nucleotides, lipid and amino acids. As T lymphocytes begin to proliferate, they also undergo differentiation into functional subsets which determine the nature of the immune response [5, 6].

The CD4+ T cells differentiate into T effector cells (Teff), including helper Th1, Th2, Th9 and Th17, follicular Tfh and Treg cells. Of these, the Th1 cells mediate responses to extracellular bacteria and helminths, Th9 cells play a role in the pathogenesis of asthma and resolution of parasitic infections, Th17 cells are important for anti-fungal defense and inflammation and Tfh cells are specialized for B cell helper. The other type of T cells is T reg cells which are asscoiated with the suppression of T cell activation [5, 6].

The predominant metabolic program in Treg cells is mitochondrial-dependent oxidation of lipid and other metabolites. On the other hand, increased aerobic glycolysis is observed in Th1, Th2, and Th17 cells. In these cells, partial activation of PI3K/Akt/mTOR pathways is also observed. Also, the transcription factor HIF1 (hypoxia inducible factor 1) has been observed as a key regulator of the anabolic metabolism in differentiating Th17 cells [5, 6].

Like CD4+ T cells, activated CD8+ T cells also switch from fatty acid oxidation to aerobic glycolysis, and shift from glycolysis to lipid oxidation once they produce CD8 memory T cells. At the end of the immune response, T cells no longer require rapid growth and therefore their glycolytic metabolism decreases. At this stage, both CD4 and CD8 T cells transform into memory T cells. Memory T cells have the ability to revert oxidation of lipids for primary energy source. This type of metabolic transition helps antigen-specific T cell clones to rapidly expand competitive selection of high affinity clones [5, 6].

Unlike T lymphocytes, activated B lymphocytes lead to a balanced increase in aerobic glycolysis and oxygen consumption [5, 6].

In addition to the cells of the adaptive immune system, cells of the innate immune system, such as dendritic cells (DC) and macrophages which are the first-line effector cells, show a metabolic switch to aerobic glycolysis. Aerobic glycolysis provides building blocks for the biosynthesis of macromolecules, such as lipids which is required for a proper balance between uptake and synthesis for immunogenicity of DCs [5, 6].

Macrophages are functionally plastic cells and are capable of tightly coordinating their metabolic programs with the functional properties. Like T cells subsets, macrophages can be associated with multiple phenotypes. The classic inflammatory macrophage is termed M1, whereas M2 macrophages are immune regulatory and immune-suppressive and also known as tumor associated macrophage (TAMs). The M1 macrophages in response to a rapid inflammatory response co-ordinately engage aerobic glycolysis, pentose phosphate shunt (PPP), glutamine and arginine catabolism to produce nitric oxide (NO) and reactive oxygen species (ROS). On the other hand, the M2 macrophages are pro-tumoral and dominant in adipose tissues of lean individuals. It produces inflammatory cytokines, such as IL-10 to maintain metabolic homeostasis through active insulin signaling. The M2 macrophages largely utilize lipid oxidation and shift arginine catabolism from iNOS mediated production of NO to produce urea and ornithine.

In other words, the M1 phenotype is glycolytic, whereas, the M2 phenotype relies on AMPK and is oxidative [5, 6].

Another class of cells, the myeloid derived suppressor cells (MDSC) show heightened glycolysis with reduced immunosuppressive function. However, the metabolic regulation in natural killer (NK) cells and neutrophils are largely unknown [5, 6].

Both cancer cells and T cells experience similar type of stressors such as: (i) rapid proliferation, (ii) synthesis of large amounts of effector proteins and (iii) entrance into heterogeneous and potentially hypoxic, nutrient poor environment. Each of these stressors has a significant link to the metabolic pathways. These similarities to meet the metabolic demand and stresses indicate that both the cancer cells and T lymphocytes adopt similar metabolic profile. However, there are differences between T cell proliferation and cancer cell proliferation. T cells change from naïve to the active T cells which are metabolically flexible and not fixed to a specific metabolic program. This is because T cells differentiate into effector, regulatory and memory T cells and their metabolism is dependent on signaling pathways triggered by the local environment. Accordingly, lipid-dependent regulatory T cells can be redirected to form highly glycolytic, IL-17 producing cells by altering the cytokine environment. On the other hand, tumor cells show fixed metabolic route which in many cases is caused by irreversible mutation of specific genes of the upstream signaling pathways or directly through the metabolic pathway genes. In addition, different cancer cells, even within the same tumor are metabolically diverse. In breast cancer and prostate cancer, this heterogeneity is considered as representative of cancer stage or subtype [7].

In addition, a major difference between activated T cell and cancer cell is that following clearance of an infection, the vast majority of T cells apoptosis is due to activation-induced cell death or programmed cell death (PCD) or cytokine neglect. Interestingly, both activated T cells and tumor cells are kept alive by a balance maintained at the pro- and anti-apoptotic BH3 domain-containing proteins. For example, in lymphocytes, this balance is maintained by cytokine signaling through Akt and other pathways and by glycolytic flux. In tumors, this balance is maintained by glycolytic flux and oncogenic signaling [8].

METABOLIC REPROGRAMMING AND IMMUNE SUPPRESSION IN TUMOR MICROENVIRONMENT

Tumor microenvironment represents a highly dynamic environment with different types of cells including immunosuppressive cells, such as myeloid-derived suppressor cells (MDSC) and regulatory T (Treg) cells. In addition, tumor associated macrophages (TAMs) within the tumor microenvironment also consist of multiple distinct pro- and anti-tumoral subpopulations. In the presence of these different types of cells, tumor cells compete for nutrients. This requires the establishement of symbiosis with the surrounding cells to meet the energy demand and cope with its high proliferation rate. Studies showed that amino acids, lactic acid and lipids derived from stromal cells, adipocytes, epithelial cells, mesenchymal stem cells or even the tumor cells from hypoxic regions can modulate tumor cell growth in response to therapy. While Otto Warbug described the existence of altered metabolic pathways in cancer cells, subsequent research on tumor metabolism and tumor immunity showed that although certain metabolites (*e.g.*, lactic acid) play immune suppressive role, oncogenes or mutation in tumor suppressor genes can also lead to immune suppression. On the other hand, certain cytokines (*e.g.*, leptin) promote tumor progression and are also associated with immune suppression in tumor microenvironment. These indicate that immune-modulation in tumor microenvironment can be multifactorial and involve components of the metabolic pathway directly or indirectly (Table 1). In this section, we will discuss metabolic reprogramming in tumor cells in the context of metabolites originating from cellular metabolism but possessing immunesuppressive role; cytokines involved in immuno suppressive role; and cell signaling pathways associated with immunosuppressive role in cancer cells [9].

Table 1. Immunosuppressive factors produced by human tumors [10].

Factors	Effect on immune system
1). TNF family ligands: FasL TRAIL TNF	Induce leukocyte apoptosis *via* the TNF family receptors

(Table 1) contd.....

Factors	Effect on immune system
2). Small molecules i) Inflammatory mediators: Prostagladin E2 (PGE2) ii) Histamine iii) Epinephrine iv) Glucose metabolism: Lactic acid v) Arginine metabolism: iNOS vi) Mitochondrial respiration: H2O2	(i)-(iii) Inhibit leukocyte functions through increased cAMP. (iv) Inhibits CTL (v) Promotes or inhibits Fas-mediated apoptosis by regulation of NO levels. (vi) Has pro-oxidant activity, increases cAMP levels, causes apoptosis in NK cells, inhibits tumor specific CTL.
3). Enzymes: i) Indoleamine 2,3-dioxygeanse (IDO) ii) Arginase I	(i) Suppresses T-cell response (ii) Impairs T-cell function, decreases ζ chain expression
4). Cytokines (i) TGF-β (ii) IL-10 (iii) GM-CSF (iv) Leptin	(i) Inhibits perforin and granzyme mRNA expression, inhibits lymphocyte proliferation. (ii) Inhibits production of IL-1β, IFN-γ, IL-12 and TNFα. (iii) Promotes expansion of immunosuppressive tumor-associated macrophages. (iv) Reduces cell apoptosis by stimulation of NF-κB signaling.
5). Tumor associated gangliosides	Inhibit IL-2 dependent lymphocyte proliferation or induce apoptotic signals.

METABOLITES ORIGINATING FROM CELLULAR METABOLISM

Glucose Metabolism

Glucose serves as energy source in normal cells. Under normoxic/aerobic condition, one mole of glucose is converted into two moles of pyruvate and two moles of NADH+H+ with a net gain of two ATPs. The pyruvate then enters the mitochondria and decarboxylated into acetyl-CoA by pyruvate dehydrogenase (PDH). However, tumor cell metabolism tends to avoid mitochondrial activity and oxidative phosphorylation (OXPHOS) and largely depends on glycolysis for ATP generation. Avoiding the mitochondrial respiration or hypoxic condition catabolizes glucose into lactic acid. Tumors cells show excessive glucose uptake rate and increased glycolytic metabolism. They obtain majority of their energy by glycolysis and maintains elevated rates of lactic acid production. Since normal mitochondrial respiration cannot occur without oxygen, hypoxia causes tumor metabolism to shift to glycolysis. As a result tumor cells require increased glucose uptake to meet their energy demand. In this context, higher expression of glucose transporter-1 (GLUT-1), lactate dehydrogenase (LDH) and monocarboxylate transporter 4(MCT4) involved in lactic acid transport are reported to be induced [11].

The high levels of lactic acid accumulation increases extracellular acidification in tumor microenvironment. Therefore, the Na^+/H^+ exchanger, the H^+ lactate co-transporter, monocarboxylate transporters (MCTs) and the proton pump (H^+-ATPase) are activated in cancer cells and play essential role in modulating the pH and ionic compositions in tumor microenvironment [11].

High levels of lactic acid have been shown to correlate with distant metastasis. Lactic acid also induced random migration of cancer cells. Lactic acid induces other factors for tumor progression. CD44, hyaluronic acid and transforming growth factor (TGF)-beta are induced by lactic acid. Furthermore, high lactic acid concentration is positively correlated with radio- resistance. Lactic acid accumulation increases acidosis in the tumor environment. Low pH increases local acidification and has positive effect on extracellular matrix degradation. Acidic pH elevates IL-8 and VEGF expressions which are important pro-angiogenic factors involved in metastasis in different cancer types. Acidic microenvironment also impairs natural killer (NK) cells by restricting IFN-gamma, IL-10 and TGF-beta. These provide evidence for lactic acid being an important source of tumor progression and metastasis [1, 11].

In addition to the direct effects of lactic acid on tumor cells in tumor progression and metastasis, it has an important impact on tumor infiltrating immune cells. Tumor derived lactic acid strongly inhibits the differentiation and activation of monocyte-derived dendritic cells *in vitro*. Dendritic cells generated in the presence of lactic acid expressed low levels of maturation-associated antigens, such as CD80, CD86 and HLA-DR and secreted less IL-12. Inhibitory effect of lactic acid on TNF secretion was also observed in human monocytes. Although these are the examples of inhibitory effect of lactic acid, it has positive effects on cytokine production, IL-23 which is involved in tumor associated inflammation and lack of tumor immunosurveillance. Pre-incubation of macrophages with sodium lactate increased the secretion of inflammatory cytokines like IL-6 and IL-8 [1, 11].

In addition to the myeloid cells, lactic acid shows modulatory effect for T lymphocytes in tumor microenvironment. Lactic acid shows strong inhibitory effect on functional properties of human T cells. It inhibits proliferation and cytokine production of human cytotoxic T lymphocytes (CTL) and decreases their cytotoxic activity [1, 11].

Arginine Metabolism

L-arginine is a non-essential amino acid and is the substrate for four enzymes in mammalian system. These are nitric oxide synthases (NOS1, NOS2, and NOS3), arginases (arginase I and II), arginine:glycine amidinotransferases (AGAT), and L-arg decarboxylase (ADC). Dietary L-arg is taken up by intestinal epithelial cells and moves across the plasma membrane *via* the catioinc amino acid transporters (CAT). Inside the cell, L-arg is metabolized by NOS enzymes producing citrulline and nitric oxide. Of these, nitric oxide plays an important role in cytotoxic mechanisms as vasodilation. On the other hand, arginase I and II metabolize L-arg to L-ornithine and urea. Of these, L-ornithine is the precursor for the production of polyamines essential for cell proliferation, whereas urea is important for detoxification of protein degradation. ADC converts L-arg to agmatine. Agmatine is then converted to putrescine and urea by agmatinase. While ADC and AGAT are less involved in the immune response, the remaining enzymes, arginase I and NOS2 in murine macrophages are differentially regulated by Th1 (IL-12, IFNγ) and Th2 (IL-4, IL-10, IL-13, TGF-β) cytokines (Fig. **1**). Studies showed that stimulation of murine macrophages with IFN-gamma regulates NOS2 exclusively, while IL-4, IL-10 and IL-13 induce arginase I. However, the mitochondrial isoform arginase II is not significantly modulated by Th1 or Th2 cytokines. The inhibition of arginase I leads to an increased expression of NOS2 which finally leads to the production of NO. Conversely, upregulation of arginase I inhibits NOS activity and contributes to the pathophysiology of several diseases, such as vascular dysfunction and asthma [12].

The mechanism of inhibition of NOS2 expression by arginase I is mediated by L-Arg depletion, which blocks the translation of NOS2. Low levels of NO also induce nitrosylation of cysteine residues of arginase I, which increases the biological activity of arginase I and further reduction at the level of L-Arg [2].

Th1 cytokines
(IL-12, INFγ)

↓

NOS

NO+Citruline

L-Arginine

Arginase I

↑

Urea+ Ornithine

Th2 cytokines (IL-4,
IL-10, IL-13, TGFβ)

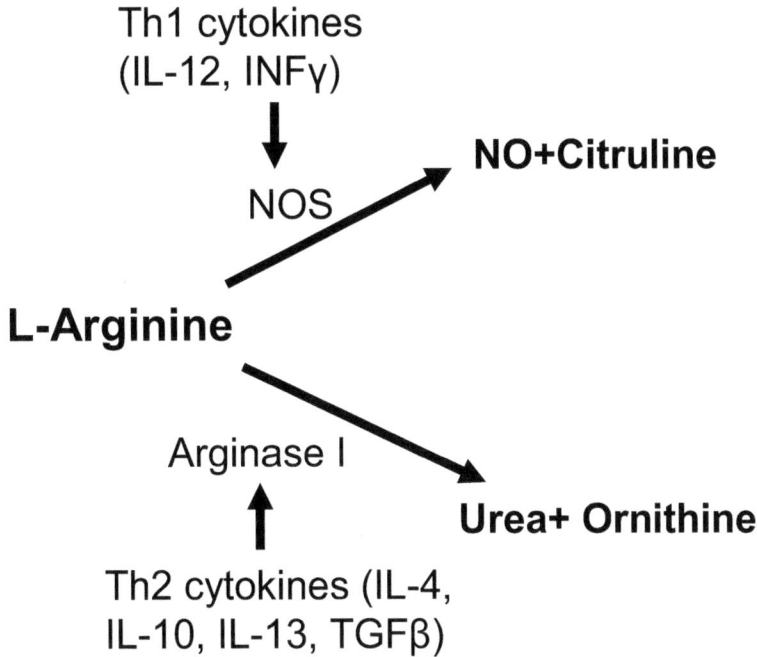

Fig. (1). Arginine metabolism and associated immune responses.

In addition, activation of murine macrophages with Th1 and Th2 has different effects on the extra-cellular levels of L-Arg, where peritoneal macrophages stimulated with IL-4 plus IL-13 increased the expression of arginase I and cationic amino acid transporter 2B (CAT-2B), leading to a rapid increase in the uptake of extracellular L-Arg with the consequent reduction of L-Arg in the microenvironment. On the other hand, macrophages stimulated with IFN-γ preferentially express NOS2 but do not increase CAT-2B and no depletion of L-Arg from the microenvironment was observed. Other than these effects, knockdown of arginase I and arginase II in mice showed that only arginase I is able to deplete serum levels of L-arginine and caused prolonged loss of CD3ζ and inhibited T cell proliferation [12, 13].

The association of L-Arg metabolism and T cell responses was observed by experiments where T cells were grown in tissue culture medium with L-Arg at different levels. L arginine levels <50μM resulted in significant decrease in cell proliferation, and decreased expression of CD3ζ, an inability to upregulate Jak-3 and decrease translocation of NFκ-B-p65. T cells cultured in the absence of L-Arg increased production of IL-2, as well as expression of early activation markers CD25, CD69, CD122 and CD132. The absence of L-Arg also arrests the Go-G1 phase of the cell cycle in activated T cells [12, 13].

Cells cultured with L-Arg progress into the S and G2-M phases. It is known that association of D-type cyclins (cyclin D1, D2 and D3), cyclin-dependent kinase 4 (cdk4) and cdk6 regulate the progression of T cells through early G1 and later into the S phase of the cell cycle. T cells cultured in the absence of L-Arg are unable to upregulate cyclin D3 and cdk4, but increases cdk6 expression. Silencing of cyclin D3 was also observed in T cells in the absence of L-Arg. L-Arg starvation also impaired the expression of cyclin D3 and cdk4 in T cells through a decreased mRNA stability and diminished translational rate. It is known that amino acid starvation impairs global translation. Accumulation of empty aminoacyl tRNAs causes amino acid starvation and activates GCN2 kinase. GCN2 kinase is known to phosphorylate the initiation factor eIF2α. The phosphorylated form of eIF2α binds with high affinity to eIF2β and blocks the exchange of GDP with GTP. This inhibits the binding of the eIF2 complex to methionine aminoacyl tRNA, decreasing the initiation of global protein synthesis. Research showed that T cells cultured in the absence of L-Arg display a decrease in global translation which is associated with higher levels of phosphor-eIF2α. The global decrease in translation impairs the expression of RNA-binding protein HuR, which inhibits mRNA stability of mRNA containing AUUA rich elements [12, 13].

Although several tumor cell lines such as non-small lung carcinoma and breast carcinoma express arginase I, this enzyme is preferentially expressed in MDSC infiltrating tumors, which inhibit T cell function and represent a possible mechanism of tumor evasion. However, it is reported that MDSC initially accumulate to fight tumors, but their phenotype changes as the tumor progresses and establishes inflammation, indicating the role of timing in this phenomenon. Furthermore, although human MDSC express high levels of arginase I, this is not upregulated by cytokines or other signals. Instead, arginase I stored in primary or gelatinase granules is released from the tumor microenvironment which significantly decreases L-arg levels, impairs T cell function and CD3delta chain expression. In fact, the release of arginase I not only leads to metabolic effect and depletion of L-arg, but also causes negative effect on the T cell response [12, 13].

Tryptophan Metabolism

Indoleamine 2,3-dioxygenase (IDO) is a tryptophan catabolizing enzyme and is overxpressed in many cancers such as melanoma, colon and RCC. IDO catalyzes the conversion of tryptophan to kynurenine and is the first enzyme in this pathway to generate nicotinamide adenine nucleotide (NAD). NAD is an important cofactor for several energy producing catabolic reactions that are involved in transcriptional regulation [10].

IDO is not only overexpressed in tumors, but also highly expressed in endothelial cells and fibroblasts. IDO leads to T cell tolerance. Overexpression of IDO in macrophages and dendritic cells creates a tolerogenic milieu *via* direct suppression of T cells and enhancement of local immunosuppression by regulatory T cells [10].

Reactive Oxygen Species

Reactive oxygen species (ROS) are radicals, ions or molecules that are generated at elevated levels in almost every cancer cells. These are ions or molecules that have a single unpaired electron in their outermost shell of electrons which make them highly reactive. ROS are categorized into two groups: free oxygen radicals and non-radical ROS. The free oxygen radicals include: superoxide (O_2^-), hydroxyl radical ($\cdot OH$), nitric oxide ($NO\cdot$), organic radicals ($R\cdot$), peroxyl radicals ($ROO\cdot$), alkoxyl radicals ($RO\cdot$), thiol radicals ($RS\cdot$), sulfonyl radicals ($ROS\cdot$), thiyl peroxyl radicals ($RSOO\cdot$), and disulfides ($RSSR$). The non-radical ROS include: hydrogen peroxide (H_2O_2), singlet oxygen ($^1O_2$), ozone/trioxygen (O3), organic hydroperoxides (ROOH), hypochloride (HOC^l), peroxynitrite (ONO−), nitroso peroxy carbonate anion ($O{=}NOOCO^2$ −), nitrocarbonate anion (O_2NOCO_2-), dinitrogen dioxide (N_2O_2), nitronium (NO^{2+}), and highly reactive lipid-or carbohydrate derived carbonyl compounds. Among the different types of ROS, superoxide, hydrogen peroxide and hydroxyl radicals are the most well studied ROS in cancer [14, 15].

At the cellular level, oxygen is required for the generation of energy during the aerobic respiration process. In eukaryotes, this takes place in the inner mitochondrial membrane where oxygen is invariably used as the terminal electron acceptor where high energy electrons from nicotinamide adenine dinucleotide (NADH) and flavin adenine dinucleotide (FADH) are transferred to oxygen *via* various electron carriers. In this way, a proton gradient is created that drives the synthesis of ATP. This eventually generates toxic free radicals *via* the reduction of oxygen to free superoxide radicals ($O2^-$) which occurs primarily within the mitochondria. It has been speculated that 1-2% of daily consumed oxygen is converted to $O2^-$ by mitochondrial respiration and upto nine of the various mitochondrial enzymes and redox carriers have been reported as possible $O2^-$ producing sites. While this is just one example of the synthesis of the superoxide radical ($O2^-$) which is a ROS, other ROS are produced in response to multiple stimuli including immunoglobulins and the T-cell receptors (TCRs) [14, 15].

However, cellular defense mechanisms exist to maintain the cellular redox in the reduced state. The antioxidant system consists of enzyme and non-enzyme molecules. Among the enzyme molecules: superoxide dismutase (SOD), catalase, glutathione peroxidase are mentionable. Among the non-enzyme molecules, glutathione (GSH), vitamin C or L-ascorbic acid, vitamin E, carotenoids and selenium are mentionable [14, 15].

Cancer cells show high levels of reactive oxygen species resulting from increased metabolic activity, mitochondrial dysfunction, peroxisome activity, increased cellular receptor signaling, oncogene activity, increased activity of oxidases, cyclooxygenases, lipooxigenases and thymidine phopsphorylase. Several growth factors and cytokines also stimulate the production of ROS to exert their diverse biological effects in cancer. Elevated levels of hydrogen peroxide and nitrite oxide were detected in tumor cells in response to interferon gamma (IFN-γ) and TNF-α. In addiiton, platelet derived growth factor (PDGF), epidermal growth factor (EGF), insulin, transforming growth factor β (TGF-β), interleukin-1 (IL-1), tumor necrosis factor alpha (TNF-α), angiotensin and lysophosphatidic acid also induce the formation of superoxidse. Even the activation of the small RhoGTPase K-ras downstream of growth factors or its oncogenic mutation increases superoxide induction and the incidences of various cancers. Depending on the cellular system, growth factors and mutant K-ras elevate intracellular superoxide levels

NADPH oxidase or mitochondria. ROS is also induced by the immunological systems in cancer [14, 15].

Macrophages induce the generation of ROS within tumor cells through the secretion of TNFalpha. Macrophages and neutrophils produce ROS to kill tumor cells. During inflammation process, macrophages generate nitric oxide which reacts with superoxide radicals and contributes to tumor cell apoptosis. However, ROS in cancer increases cell cycle progression and proliferation, cell survival and energy metabolism, cell morphology, cell-cell adhesion, cell motility, angiogenesis and maintenance of tumor stemness. Low doses of hydrogen peroxide and superoxide stimulate cell proliferation in different types of cancer cells. For example, decreased MnSOD activity has been reported in breast cancer cells favoring proliferation of the cells and increased superoxide and low hydrogen peroxide levels. Increased MnSOD activity drives the proliferating cells to transit to quiescent states due to increased generation of hydrogen peroxide [14, 15].

Reactive oxygen species also regulates cell cycle progression. It upregulates the mRNA levels of cyclins which participate in the progression of cell cycle from G1 to S phase transition including cyclin B2, cyclin D3, cyclin E1 and cyclin E2. An environemental carcinogen sodium arsenite stimulates ROS production in breast cancer cells and potentiates S phase progression and subsequent cell proliferation [14, 15].

Elevated levels of ROS are also known to contribute to tumorigenesis and metastasis by triggering signals related to angiogenesis. ROS mediates activation of c-met which is an HGF receptor and involved in metastasis and abnormal NF-κB activity in a number of cancers. NADPH oxidase derived ROS from macrophages and neutrophils contributes to the upregulation of thymosin-beta 4 gene which plays a vital role in tumor cell motility and invasiveness. While these are some of the examples on the role of ROS in tumorgenesis and metastasis, the major contributors to ROS pool in cancer are myeloid cells [14, 15].

The myeloid cells include granulocytes, macrophages and myeloid derived suppressor cells (MDSC). The later cells are present in the majority of cancer patients. MDSCs usually include two major subpopulations: monocytic MDSCs (M-MDSCs) and granulocytic MDSCs (G-MDSCs). In humans, MDSCs constitute a heterogenous cell population that are not well characterized due to the absence of unified markers. However, some of these cells express the common myeloid markers such as CD33 and CD11b but lacks mature myeloid cells such as HLA-DR. In addition, the monocytic subset comprises of CD14+ cells and the granulocytic subset comprises of CD14-CD15+ cells. MDSCs inhibit anti-tumor immunity by suppressing T cell and NK cell functions by increasing the production of arginine, reactive oxygen species (ROS) and nitric oxide (NO) and by inducing Treg cells and TGF-beta secretion to mediate T cell suppression [14, 15].

The suppression of immune responses by MDSC is partially mediated by loss or significant decrease of the expression of T-cell receptor ζ chain (CD3ζ) which is the principal part of TCR complex, inhibition of CD3/CD28-induced T-cell activation/proliferation by production of reactive nitrogen and oxygen intermediates, and inhibition of interferon- γ (IFN-γ) production by CD8+ T cells in response to the specific peptide presented by MHC class I molecules and prevention of the development of CTL *in vitro*. Since most MDSC effects on T cells require close cell-cell contact and depend on MHC expression by MDSC, the subset of MDSC expressing Gr-1+CD115+ cells suppresses T-cell proliferation and induces the development of Foxp3+ Tregs *in vivo*. Gr-1+ MDSC is differentiated into F4/80+ macrophages where inside tumor these macrophages produce high levels of nitric oxide and induce T-cell apoptosis. The Treg cells require antigen associated activation of tumor-specific T cells and are dependent on the presence of IFN-γ and IL-10. This interaction is independent of nitric oxide availability. While nitric oxide is required for suppression of mitogen-activated T cells by MDSC, the inhibition of allogenic T-cell responses by MDSC was mediated by enzyme arginase-1 [14, 15].

We mentioned earlier that MDSC express the common myeloid marker CD33 but lack the expression of markers of mature myeloid and lymphoid cells and HLA-DR or CD14-CD11b+ cells. Studies showed that in case of advanced stage cancer, there is accumulation of these cells in blood, whereas the surgical resection of the tumor decreased the number of immature cells. Blood samples from cancer patients showed an unusually large number of myeloid cells with granulocyte phenotype. These cells can inhibit cytokine production by T cells. Of the different types of ROS mentioned above, peroxynitrite is one of the most powerful reactive oxidant species, which is responsible for most of the adverse effects linked with ROS. Peroxynitrite is a product of reaction of nitric oxide (NO) and superoxide (O2.-). Nitric oxide produced by macrophages inhibits T cells *via* a variety of different mechanisms. Mentionables are: inhibition of the phosphorylation and activation of Janus kinase 3 (Jak3) and STAT5 transcription factor, (ii) inhibition of MHC class II gene expression and (iii) induction of T-cell apoptosis. Peroxynitrites inhibit T-cell activation and proliferation *via* impairment of tyrosine phosphorylation and apoptotic death, and also cause nitration of proteins involved in the removal of oxidatively modified proteins [14, 15].

Peroxynitrites produced during inflammatory conditions can modify and inactivate proteins, especially zinc finger transcription factors, such as p53. Peroxynitrite is also involved in MDSC mediated T-cell tolerance. During antigen presentation, MDSC closely interacts with antigen specific T cells. This interaction can be affected by the abundance of peroxynitrite. For example, tumor-derived factors stimulate production and activation of MDSC that contain high levels of ROS and generate peroxynitrite. Since MDSC accumulate in the lymph nodes of tumor bearing host and ROS are short-lived and highly reactogenic, these are capable of acting only in short distance. Therefore, interface of MDSC and CD8+ T cells interacting during antigen-TCR recognition phase leads peroxynitrite to produce nitrate tyrosine residues, exposed on the surface of contacting cells. Modified tyrosine on TCR and CD8 alters the conformational flexibility of TCR chain and loses the response to specific antigen [14, 15].

MDSC also migrate into tumor site where they differentiate into tumor-associated macrophages (TAM). Tumor microenvironment downregulates ROS production and induces iNOS expression *via* upregulation of STAT1. TAM produces high levels of NO and immunosuppressive cytokines (*e.g.*, IL-10). These create immunosuppressive environment where T-cell function is inhibited in antigen non-specific manner [14, 15].

The role of ROS in tumor development and progression has considerable importance as this leads to alterations in nucleic acid structure and inhibition of repair enzymes, where ROS contributes to the accumulation of genomic abnormalities leading to malignant transformation of cells. ROS not only blocks the activation of caspases, which lead to the inhibition of apoptosis, but also inhibits immune responses in cancer *via* various mechanisms involving direct effect on T-cell receptors, such as blocking of signal transduction and affecting gene transcription. Peroxynitrite is involved in ROS-mediated immune suppression, blocks its generation or use its scavengers which could decrease or eliminate MDSC-induced T-cell tolerance and enhance the effect of cancer immunotherapy [14, 15].

Cytokines Associated with Tumor Progression

Leptin

Leptins are adipocyte-derived hormone or cytokines. They control food intake and energy expenditure in humans. Circulating leptin reflects host metabolic/ nutritional status. Leptin also modulates Treg cell function. In this way, it links external/environmental signals or nutrient availability with regulation of T cell tolerance [16].

Leptin is a product of the obese (*ob*) gene with a molecular weight of 16 kDa. Leptin mRNA is primarily detected in white and brown adipose tissues. However, leptin is also synthesized by non-adipose tissues. Other sources of leptin include gastric mucosa cells, mammary epithelial cells, myocytes, placenta, testes, ovary and hair follicles [16].

Primary function of leptin is to act as the regulator of body weight and energy balance in the hypothalamus. However, leptin can also affect fetal development, sex maturation, lactation, hematopoiesis, and immune responses [16].

In humans, the major factor influencing plasma leptin concentrations is adipose tissue mass. Circulating leptin levels exhibit strong positive correlation with total body fat, and to a lesser degree with BMI (body mass index). Serum leptin concentration is high in women than man. This indicates the differential regulation of leptin expression by sex hormones, with estrogens reported to upregulate and testosterone is observed to decrease leptin levels. The synthesis of leptin in adipocytes is influenced by different humoral factors, such as insulin, melanoyl-CoA, ATP, glucosamine and short chain fatty acids. Its expression is inhibited by cyclic AMP, testosterone and long-chain fatty acid. Leptin expression is also induced by different inflammatory immune mediators, such as tumor necrosis factor alpha (TNF-α), glucocorticoids and prostaglandins, some of which have been associated with neoplastic processes. Under normal conditions, the levels of circulating leptin correlate positively with the leptin mRNA and protein levels in adipose tissue, however, the levels of leptin rapidly increases during acute infection and sepsis [16].

In the context of cancer, both hypoxia and chemicals inducing cellular hypoxia are able to activate the leptin gene promoter through the hypoxia-induced factor-1 (HIF-1) in human adipocytes and fibroblasts. Leptin regulates neoangiogenesis by itself and in concert with vascular endothelial growth factor (VEGF) and fibroblast growth factor (FGF) 2. Leptin can also enhance endothelial cell growth and suppress apoptosis through a Bcl-2 dependent mechanism. In addition, leptin can increase the levels and activity of enzymes involved in angiogenesis, such as matrix metalloproteinases (MMPs) 2 and 9. Leptin also acts as a mitogen, transforming factor, or migration factor for many different cell types including smooth muscle cells, normal and neoplastic colon cells, normal and malignant mammary epithelial cells [16].

The activities of leptin are mediated through the transmembrane leptin receptor, ObR, which belongs to the class I cytokine receptor family including receptors for IL-2, IL-6, G-CSF, LIF, CNTF, OSM and gp130. By alternative splicing, OB-R mRNA gives rise to six different isoforms. While all the ObR share identical extracellular binding domain, the cytoplasmic domains differ in length. The full form of ObR is 1,165 amino acids long and contains the extracellular, transmembrane and intracellular domain. The extracellular domain binds ligand, whereas the intracellular tail recruits and activates signaling substrates. Of the four isoforms, only ObR1 contains an active intracellular signaling domain and has the ability to activate intracellular JAK2-STAT, Ras-ERK1/2 and PI3K-Ak--GSK3 pathways. ObR1 is highly expressed in the hypothalamus, however, lower levels of ObR1 has been identified in many peripheral organs. On the other hand, short (Ob-Rs/Ra) isoforms lack major domains and mainly activate MAPK and have little effect on STAT activation [16].

In addition to signal transduction pathways, the role of leptin in innate immunity has been demonstrated by a wide range of leptin actions on antigen-presenting cells (APCs), natural killer cells (NK) and neutrophils. Leptin expression can be induced by inflammatory stimuli, such as LPS, IL-1 and TNF-alpha during acute phase of immune response. These indicate that leptin act as mediator in regulating inflammatory activities. Leptin signaling has been associated with the maturation and survival of DC. Leptin also stimulates proliferation and phagocytosis in monocytes and macrophages. In macrophages, leptin induces factors are found to be involved in regulating immune responses, such as nitric oxide, leukotriene B4 (LTB4), cholesterol acyl-transferase-1 (ACAT-1) and cyclooxygenase 2 (COX-2). Leptin induces the production of growth hormone by protein kinase C (PKC) and nitric oxide-dependent pathways in peripheral blood mononuclear cells. Overall, leptin plays pleiotropic role in maintaining immune homeostasis by regulating the survival and activity of immune cells of the innate immune response [17].

Since leptin can stimulate pro-inflammatory cytokine production involving the innate immune response, these can indirectly modulate the adaptive immune system. For example, the leptin-induced type I cytokines such as IL-12 and TNF-α in DC can prime CD4$^+$ Th1 cells. Leptin also plays a direct role in adaptive immunity by modulating T-cell mediated immune responses. Furthermore, leptin promotes survival of T and B lymphocytes by suppressing Fas-mediated apoptosis [17].

While the immunomodulatory role of leptin in immunity has become increasingly evident, the other major function of leptin as an endocrine hormone to regulate energy storage and metabolism has added complexity in ascertaining the role of leptin either in immune modulation or in metabolic functions. Despite this controversy, leptin expression has been reported to be upregulated in many types of cancers such as breast cancer, colorectal cancer *etc.* [17].

In the context of cancer, *in vitro* studies in breast cancer cell models showed that leptin increased cell proliferation, cell transformation, and activation of the

ERK1/2, STAT3, Akt/GSK3, and PKC-alpha pathways. Leptin also increased AP-1 activation, upregulation of cdk2, cyclin D1, hyperphosphorylation of pRb, induced expression of *c-myc* and stabilization of ERα expression [17].

In colorectal cancer, leptin increased cell invasion *via* PI-3K, Rho- and Rac-dependent pathway. It also increased cell growth through the ERK1/2 pathway and reduced cell apoptosis stimulation of NF-κB signaling [17].

In prostate cancer leptin increased cell proliferation and suppressed apoptosis. On the other hand, in pancreatic cancer, leptin decreased cell proliferation and stimulated STAT3 and STAT5b phosphorylation. Furthermore, in ovarian cancer, leptin increased proliferation *via* the ERK1/2 pathway. In lung cancer also, leptin stimulated cell proliferation *via* the ERK1/2 pathway. In addition to the solid tumors, ObR1 and ObRs mRNAs have been detected in several myeloid and lymphoid leukemic cell lines, where the hormone stimulated the proliferation of human myeloid leukemic cell lines. Leptin in combination with other hematopoietic cytokines (IL-3, G-CSF, and SCF) induced an additive or synergistic mitogenic response in several acute myeloid leukemia (AML) cases. In addition to *in vitro* studies, elevated levels of serum leptin have been detected in breast cancer, colorectal cancer (in men but not in women), prostate cancer, pancreatic cancer *etc.* [16 - 18].

Both *in vivo* and *in vitro* studies indicate that serum leptin concentrations are critical for tumor progression and leptin abundance in tumor environment can be regulated by surrounding adipose tissue. In addition, tumor cells themselves can produce the hormone. This indicates that leptin inhibiting drugs can be effective in cancer treatment and prevention [16 - 18].

Indeed there are several therapeutic approaches for interfering with leptin's action in breast cancer cell development and progression. A leptin peptide antagonist (LPA) corresponding to amino acids 70-95, inhibited tumor growth of a murine mammary cancer cell line. There have been reports of mutated leptin analogs that either function as antagonist or agonist or as both. Another approach was to develop synthetic peptides representing relevant amino acids of the leptin molecule which blocked leptin mediated signaling [19].

Signaling Pathways Associated with Tumor Progression

Autophagy Pathway

Autophagy is a highly conserved and regulated process that occurs at the basal level to control the protein level in eukaryotic cells. The process of autophagy is initiated by several factors including starvation condition or the presence of drugs such as rapamycin. There are several steps involved in this process where the damaged protein and some components of the cytoplasm are enveloped into double-membraned autophagosome vesicles that fuse with the lysosome for degradation. Previously, autophagy was thought to be a process of programmed cell death II. However, recent research shows that autophagy is also involved in tumor progression and cell survival. As a result, many autophagy genes are currently known as oncogenes instead of tumor suppressors. Details of the genes involved in this process will be discussed in chapter 3. Here we will discuss mostly the autophagy pathway genes involved in modulating innate and adaptive systems, and involvement of the autophagy pathway genes in the development of different types of cancer [20].

Autophagy is induced both by starvation condition and environmental stress responses. While starvation induced autophagy degrades cellular components in a non-specific manner, environmental stress responses induce selective autophagy. Here environmental stress response refers to the accumulation of protein aggregates, damaged organelles or intracellular bacteria and viruses. The autophagy pathway plays an important role in maintaining cellular homeostasis by organelle recycling, metabolism and host defense; it is an essential part of both the innate and adaptive immune systems. Some bacteria and virus suppress autophagy, whereas other bacteria and virus utilize autophagosome membranes and the autophagic machinery to enhance their replication [20].

Research showed that autophagy influences the adaptive immune response by functioning in the processing and delivery of microbial and viral antigens for MHC class I and II presentations. However, MHC class II antigen presentation has been reported to be associated with Epstein-Barr virus processing. Epstein Barr virus is associated with particular forms of cancer, such as Hodgkin's lymphoma, Burkitt's lymphoma and nasopharyngeal carcinoma. During MHC class II antigen presentation, exogenous peptides are processed by hydrolase enzymes present in the lysosomal compartments and are presented on the cell surface antigen-presenting cells to activate CD4+ T cell responses. Dendritic cells, B cells and epithelial cells are MHC class II-positive cells. These cells form autophagosomes that fuse with multivesicular MHC class II-loading compartments. While the Epstein Barr virus nuclear antigen protein (EBNA1) is the dominant CD4+ T cell antigen which is detected during latent Epstein-Barr virus (EBV) infection, the role of autophagy in this process has been investigated by using autophagy inhibitor 3-MA or siRNA knockdown of *Atg12*, leading to down-regulation of endogenous MHC class II processing of EBNA1 [21].

Dysregulation of the autophagy pathway has been implicated in other human cancers also. The Akt/mammalian target of rapamycin (mTOR), a serine/threonine kinase negatively regulates autophagy upstream of ULK1/2. mTOR is constitutively activated in Kaposi's sarcoma (KS) and KSHV-associated primary effusion lymphoma (PEL). Kaposi's sarcoma is a common complication following organ transplantation and administration of immunosuppressive treatment [20].

CONCLUSION

Studies showing metabolic reprogramming or altered metabolism in tumor is almost a century old. However, the importance of the complex relationship between tumor metabolism, tumor progression and immunosuppression is still under investigation. Alteration of the metabolic pathways in tumor cells represents an attractive target for the development of anti-cancer drugs. However, targeting tumor cell metabolism may not be the only approach to eliminating tumor cells. Over the past several years, small molecule inhibitors have been used to target the specific metabolic pathways in tumor cells. However, their off-target effect on the proliferating immune cells in the tumor microenvironment is also a concern to treat cancer.

The presence of tumor-reactive T-lymphocyte responses provides the basis for successful immunotherapeutic approaches against cancer. Activated T lymphocytes (*e.g.*, tumor-infiltrating lymphocytes (TILs)) play important role in eliminating malignant tumor cells. As a result, high frequencies of TILs are associated with a lower risk of relapse, reduced tumor progression and overall survival in cancer patients, particularly melanoma and colorectal cancer. Over the past two decades, different strategies to stimulate anti-tumor immunity by using therapeutic vaccination and adoptive T-cell transfer have been extensively studied. However, the immune escape mechanism of tumor cells leads to ineffectiveness of the treatment procedure. Therefore, tumor specific T cells can be genetically modified to become resistant to suppress tumor metabolites in order to enhance functional activity of T-cells. Knockdown of GCN2 tumor reactive T cells using siRNA has been shown to render T-cells resistant to IDO-induced anergy. In addition, direct inhibition of key metabolic enzymes, such as IDO, iNOS and arginase was shown to reconstitute anti-tumoral T-cell activity. Inhibition of LDHA by oxamic acid in tumor spheroids recovered T-cell effector functions *in vitro* [22].

Again increased glycolysis in cancer cells is regulated by the autophagy pathway regulators, such as Akt/mTOR and even transcription factors such as HIF1. Temsirolimus, a specific inhibitor of mTOR improved survival among patients with metastatic renal cell carcinoma. PX-478, an inhibitor of HIF1 showed remarkable anti-tumor activity *in vitro* and *in vivo*. LW6, a novel HIF-1 inhibitor promotes proteasomal degradation of HIF1α in colon cancer. Another inhibitor of HIF is bevacizumab, a monoclonal antibody that binds to circulating VEGF protein, producing significant prolongation of time to disease progression in RCC [22].

In addition, there are also inhibitors of the glycolytic pathway enzymes. 2-deoxyglucose (2DG) or ionidamine inhibit this key enzyme and augments apoptosis. Another promising drug is dichloroacetic acid (DCA) which inhibits pyruvate dehydrogenase kinase (PDK) enzyme and leads to reduction in tumor growth [22].

Metabolic profiles represent the closest phenotype of a cell. As tumor environment is a complex system it is not unusual to see transformation of the immune responsive system into the immunosuppressive system by tumor metabolites. While the consequence of these modifications not only affects the function of the therapies used to treat cancer, but reversal of the existing immune dysfunction may shed some light to design proper therapies to treat cancer. Therefore, identifying these factors will enhance our understanding on the mechanism of immunosuppression and tumor progression and also on the therapy resistance of tumor cells. In conclusion, research on tumor metabolism has significant potential to influence the adaptive immune responses for innovative anti-cancer therapies. The development of drugs that specifically modulates the altered tumor metabolism may improve targeting cancer cells and also tumor-specific T-cell responses to correct immune imbalance, deliver adequate *in vivo* stimulation, transfer effector T cells that are capable of *in vivo* expansion, and provide protection for the immune effector cell re-populating the host. Survival of these cells will have long-term memory development in patients with malignancy which is necessary for improving clinical benefits.

CONFLICT OF INTEREST

The author confirms that author has no conflict of interest to declare for this publication.

ACKNOWLEDGEMENTS

Declared none.

REFERENCES

[1]   Mesure D. Cancer metabolic and immune Reprogramming : The Intimate interaction between cancer cells and microenvironment. J Cancer Prev Curr Res 2014; 1: 1-8.

[2]   Singer K, Gottfried E, Kreutz M, Mackensen A. Suppression of T-cell responses by tumor metabolites. Cancer Immunol Immunother 2011; 60(3): 425-31.
        [http://dx.doi.org/10.1007/s00262-010-0967-1] [PMID: 21240484]

[3]   Hall CJ, Sanderson LE, Crosier KE, Crosier PS. Mitochondrial metabolism, reactive oxygen species, and macrophage function-fishing for insights. J Mol Med (Berl) 2014; 1119-28.

[4]   Ward PS, Thompson CB. Metabolic reprogramming: a cancer hallmark even warburg did not anticipate. Cancer Cell 2012; 21(3): 297-308.
        [http://dx.doi.org/10.1016/j.ccr.2012.02.014] [PMID: 22439925]

[5]   Wang T, Liu G, Wang R. The Intercellular Metabolic Interplay between Tumor and Immune Cells. Front Immunol 2014; 5: 358.
        [http://dx.doi.org/10.3389/fimmu.2014.00358] [PMID: 25120544]

[6]   Rathmell JC. Metabolism and autophagy in the immune system: immunometabolism comes of age. Immunol Rev 2012; 249(1): 5-13.
[http://dx.doi.org/10.1111/j.1600-065X.2012.01158.x] [PMID: 22889211]

[7]   Procaccini C, Galgani M, De Rosa V, Matarese G. Intracellular metabolic pathways control immune tolerance. Trends Immunol 2012; 33(1): 1-7.
[http://dx.doi.org/10.1016/j.it.2011.09.002] [PMID: 22075206]

[8]   Macintyre AN, Rathmell JC. Activated lymphocytes as a metabolic model for carcinogenesis. Cancer Metab 2013; 1(1): 5.
[http://dx.doi.org/10.1186/2049-3002-1-5] [PMID: 24280044]

[9]   Villalba M, Rathore MG, Lopez-Royuela N, Krzywinska E, Garaude J, Allende-Vega N. From tumor cell metabolism to tumor immune escape. Int J Biochem Cell Biol 2013; 45(1): 106-13.
[http://dx.doi.org/10.1016/j.biocel.2012.04.024] [PMID: 22568930]

[10]   Whiteside TL. Immune suppression in cancer: effects on immune cells, mechanisms and future therapeutic intervention. Semin Cancer Biol 2006; 16(1): 3-15.
[http://dx.doi.org/10.1016/j.semcancer.2005.07.008] [PMID: 16153857]

[11]   Dang CV. Links between metabolism and cancer. Genes Dev 2012; 26(9): 877-90.
[http://dx.doi.org/10.1101/gad.189365.112] [PMID: 22549953]

[12]   Bronte V, Serafini P, Mazzoni A, Segal DM, Zanovello P. L-arginine metabolism in myeloid cells controls T-lymphocyte functions. Trends Immunol 2003; 24(6): 302-6.
[http://dx.doi.org/10.1016/S1471-4906(03)00132-7] [PMID: 12810105]

[13]   Rodriguez PC, Quiceno DG, Ochoa AC. L-arginine availability regulates T-lymphocyte cell-cycle progression. Blood 2007; 109(4): 1568-73.
[http://dx.doi.org/10.1182/blood-2006-06-031856] [PMID: 17023580]

[14]   Adler V, Yin Z, Tew KD, Ronai Z. Role of redox potential and reactive oxygen species in stress signaling. Oncogene 1999; 18(45): 6104-11.
[http://dx.doi.org/10.1038/sj.onc.1203128] [PMID: 10557101]

[15]   Cemerski S, Cantagrel A, Van Meerwijk JP, Romagnoli P. Reactive oxygen species differentially affect T cell receptor-signaling pathways. J Biol Chem 2002; 277(22): 19585-93.
[http://dx.doi.org/10.1074/jbc.M111451200] [PMID: 11916964]

[16]   Garofalo C, Surmacz E. Leptin and cancer. J Cell Physiol 2006; 207(1): 12-22.
[http://dx.doi.org/10.1002/jcp.20472] [PMID: 16110483]

[17]   van den Brink GR, O'Toole T, Hardwick JC, *et al.* Leptin signaling in human peripheral blood mononuclear cells, activation of p38 and p42/44 mitogen-activated protein (MAP) kinase and p70 S6 kinase. Mol Cell Biol Res Commun 2000; 4(3): 144-50.
[http://dx.doi.org/10.1006/mcbr.2001.0270] [PMID: 11281728]

[18]   Lam QL, Lu L. Role of leptin in immunity. Cell Mol Immunol 2007; 4(1): 1-13.
[PMID: 17349207]

[19]   Ray A, Cleary M. Leptin as a potential therapeutic 2010; 443-51.

[20]   Virgin HW, Levine B. Autophagy genes in immunity. Nat Immunol 2009; 10(5): 461-70.

[http://dx.doi.org/10.1038/ni.1726] [PMID: 19381141]

[21]   Choi KS. Autophagy and cancer. Exp Mol Med 2012; 44(2): 109-20.
       [http://dx.doi.org/10.3858/emm.2012.44.2.033] [PMID: 22257886]

[22]   Zhang P, Zweidler-mckay PA. Notch signaling in cancer metastasis. In: Wu W-S, Hu C-T, Eds. Signal
       Transduct Cancer Metastasis. Springer Netherlands 2010; pp. 157-74.
       [http://dx.doi.org/10.1007/978-90-481-9522-0_9]

CHAPTER 3

Signal Transduction Molecules and Pathways in Cancer: Implication of the Immune System in Modulating Cancer Development and Progression

Abstract: Signal transduction pathways and associated molecules play important role in maintaining cell death and cell survival. However, in cancer cells, some of these molecules are mutated and lead to cancer progression. These molecules also interfere with the components of the humoral and the cell mediated immune systems in tumor environment. Therefore, identifying these can be potential targets for cancer treatment.

Keywords: Apoptosis, Autophagy, JAK-STAT, K-ras, Myc, p53, Signal transduction pathways.

INTRODUCTION

The tumor microenvironment consists of primary tumor and stromal cells. A variety of cell types populate the stromal compartments, which include smooth muscle cells, myofibroblasts, carcinoma associated fibroblasts, vascular cells and immune cells. Of these, vascular cells include lymph-endothelial, vascular-endothelial cells and pericytes whereas the immune cells include lymphocytes, tumor associated monocytes/macrophages (TAM) and dendritic cells. Once the tumor cells and the stromal cells interact inside the tumor microenvironment, this induces the secretion of growth factors and cytokines leading to neovasculation and modifications of the extracellular matrix (ECM), which greatly support the growth and survival of tumor cells. The onset of cancer metastasis or dissemination of the primary tumor to distant body sites is one of the most complicated processes and cancer metastasis is one of the major causes of cancer related death. Critical steps in cancer metastasis include: (i) detachment of the

Mahbuba Rahman

primary cancer cells followed by migration and invasion to adjacent tissues, (ii) penetration of the extracellular matrix (ECM) and blood vessels (intravasation), (iii) subsequent penetration out of vessels (extravasation) and (iv) proliferation in a secondary site [1].

Interestingly, not all epithelial cells are capable of expressing the metastatic phenotype. Only those that are able to escape the primary tumor and enter the circulatory system (blood or lymphatic) and break down the basement membrane allow invasion, which is critical for metastasis. The ability of the cancer cells to leave the tumor mass not only depends on losing cell-cell contact at an early stage, but it is also associated with a change in cell shape referred to as the epithelial-to-mesenchymal transition (EMT). EMT is associated with the loss of cell adhesion proteins such as E-cadherin. Once the cells are in the circulatory system, the isolated cancer cells must survive at a distant site and form a micro-colony. While the inflammatory responses within the microenvironment can be triggered by tumor hypoxia, necrosis and excessive tumor cell proliferation, the inflammatory cytokines including colony stimulating factors (CSF)-1, granulocyte- monocyte (GM-CSF), transforming growth factor (TGF)-beta, chemokines (CCL2, CCL7, CCL3, CCL4) , vascular endothelial growth factor (VEGF), IL-8, *etc.* play an important role in promoting and recruiting additional inflammatory cells such as mast cells and neutrophils to facilitate tumor progression [1, 2].

It is now well established that the association between cancer and inflammation leads to cancer development. Various pro-inflammatory mediators triggered by inflammation aid tumor progression by regulating cascades of cytokines, chemokines, adhesion and pro-angiogenic activities. Whereas chronic inflammation predisposes to cancer, neoplastic transformation predisposes to an intrinsic pro-inflammatory microenvironment which further promotes progression towards malignancy [2].

Stimuli that are associated with this transformation can be grouped into two types. The extrinsic stimuli are bacteria, viruses, non-healing wounds, irritants, *etc.* On the other hand, the intrinsic stimuli are oncogenes, protein kinases, *etc.* Both types of stimuli trigger inflammation in tumor microenvironment. For example, about

1.2 million cases of infection related malignancies are caused due to chronic inflammation induced by bacteria and virus. Viruses such as human papilloma virus, hepatitis C virus and hepatitis B virus not only inhibit tumor suppressor proteins but also cause malignancy through inflammation related mechanisms. Organs that are highly susceptible to tumor development following chronic inflammation are gastrointestinal tracts, lungs, bladder, liver, pancreas and oesophagus. On the other hand, intrinsic stimuli for inflammation are mostly the oncogenens, cytokines and even the transcription factors such as necrosis factor (NF-κB), HIF1α, STAT3, Ras-Raf signaling, MYC, *etc.* These intrinsic stimuli converge signals in the nucleus of the tumor cells and co-ordinate inflammatory transcriptional activity by activating various nuclear transcription factors mentioned above. The cross talk between these transcription factors results in a complex web of signaling processes that further promote inflammation, facilitate tumor progression, proliferation, survival and angiogenesis [2, 3].

Since the intrinsic signal transduction molecules play an important role in triggering pro-cancer inflammatory responses, in this chapter, we will discuss some of those molecules that are potential targets for cancer treatment. Signaling molecules can be single protein molecules that activate several pathways or can be transcription factors that regulate the expression of several proteins and transduce signals to the cells. However, a number of signaling pathways that play an important role in tumor regression may be involved in cancer development or progression [4].

SIGNALING MOLECULES ASSOCIATED WITH CANCER DEVELOPMENT

JAK-STAT

Cytokines like interferons (IFNs) exert their biological functions by activating genes such as Janus kinase (JAK)-signal transducer and activator of transcription (STAT) pathway, which are used by many other cytokines too. Once a cytokine binds to its cell-surface receptor, the receptor dimerizes and subsequently activates JAK tyrosine kinases, which are constitutively associated with the receptor. Specific tyrosine residues on the receptor are then phosphorylated by activated JAKS and serve as docking sites for a family of latent cytoplasmic transcription factors, which in this case are STATs. STATs are phosphorylated by JAKs and then dimerized and subsequently leave the receptor and translocate to the nucleus where they activate gene transcription. The importance of JAK-STAT pathway in cancer biology is that activation of JAK-STAT3 pathway has been repeatedly correlated with increased invasion and metastasis in a wide variety of cancer types [3, 5].

The mammalian JAK family consists of four members: JAK1, JAK2, JAK3 and tyrosine kinase 2 (TYK2). Each protein contains a conserved kinase domain and catalytically inactive, pseudo-kinase domain at the carboxyl terminus. This pseudo-kinase domain is thought to be associated in regulating the kinase activity of JAKs. However, JAK can be activated in the absence of ligand binding upon mutation of JH1 and JH2 domains [3, 5].

There are seven STAT (signal transducer and activator of transcription) mammalian proteins. These are STAT1, STAT2, STAT3, STAT4, STAT5A, STAT5B and STAT6. Of these, STAT2 is largely involved in viral infection; STATs 4 and 6 are primarily involved in lymphocyte function; STAT5A/B can promote invasion and metastasis; and STAT1 and STAT3 have been implicated in cancer progression. However, STAT1 and STAT3 play opposite roles in cancer. STAT1 is associated with anti-proliferative role, while STAT3 is associated with tumor proliferation and in promoting cell migration, invasion and metastasis [2, 3, 5].

In normal cells, STAT3 signaling is under tight regulation by the negative feedback mechanisms involving the suppressors of cytokine signaling (SOCs) and tyrosine phosphatases. But in cancer cells, STAT3 expression is constitutive and ubiquitous. STAT3 activation requires phosphorylation at tyrosine 705 location, which is achieved by growth factor receptors that have inherent tyrosine kinase activity (*c.g.*, EGFR, ERBB2, VEGFR and PDGFR) in response to growth factor stimulation. These receptors can also recruit non-receptor kinases such as SRC and ABL, which also activate STAT3. Studies showed that constitutive activation of these receptors by either their over-expression or as a result of mutation has been associated with increased invasion and metastasis in many cancer cell types.

STAT3 can also be activated by interleukin family of cytokines, but requires recruitment of kinases such as JAKs. JAKs phosphorylate tyrosine residues on the STAT, facilitating STAT3 activation and its relocation to the nucleus, leading to transcription of the target genes [2, 3, 5].

The constitutive activation of STATs in cancer cells is usually facilitated through excessive stimulation by cytokines or growth factors, which are either produced by the tumor themselves or derived from either stromal or inflammatory cells associated with tumor development or STAT3 can stimulate its own activation by regulating genes (IL-6, IL-10 and EGF) that promote its increased activation or are themselves direct STAT3 activators (*e.g.*, RAS, SRC and ABL). *In vitro* studies showed that JAK-STAT3 signaling can be activated by IL-6, which increases migration and invasion and also increases metastasis *in vivo* [2, 3, 5].

As mentioned earlier, phosphor-activation of STAT3 by JAKs is required for dimerization and functional activation of STAT3 as a transcription factor. STAT3 is known to regulate the expression of metalloproteinase (MMP) that degrades the basement membranes and extracellular matrix, which is associated with aggressive cancers and facilitates intravasation into the vasculature and extravasation at the metastatic site. STAT3 also acts as a transcription factor for several other proteins such as HSP70, HSP90, HIF1alpha, VEGFR, *etc.* indicating the bad impact of STAT3 on the expression of genes that promote invasion [2, 3, 5].

STAT3 in many human cancers also functions as a critical mediator of oncogenic signaling through transcriptional activation of genes encoding apoptosis inhibitors (*e.g.*, Bcl-xL, Mcl-1 and survivin), cell cycle regulators (*e.g.*, cyclin D1 and c-Myc) [2, 3, 5].

Overall, it is indicated that STAT3 has a central role in regulating cancer-associated inflammation by controlling the expression of various inflammatory modulators and oncogenes. A number of inhibitors of STAT3 are in use in preclinical trials [2, 3, 5].

Since STAT3 is associated with tumor growth factors and angiogenesis, the inhibitory or immunosuppression mechanism of STAT3 needs to be understood to develop drugs against STAT3 [6].

STAT3 mediated immunosuppression occurs at the inhibition of Th1 immune response, cytokine associated immune response and signaling and immunosuppression of the myeloid derived suppressor cells. STAT3 as a negative regulator of Th1 immune system was observed by increased production of Th1 cytokines such as IFNγ, TNFα and IL-1 under the ablation of STAT3 in neutrophils and macrophages and in the presence of LPS stimulation. Other than inhibiting the Th1 immune response, STAT3 promotes expansion of tumor myeloid derived suppressor cells (MDSC), which inhibit CD4+ and CD8+ T cell activation [6].

A number of factors that are involved in signaling MDSC cell expansion include IL-1β, IL-6, VEGF, COX2 and GM-CSF. Exposure of myeloid cells to tumor cell conditioned medium upregulated STAT3 activity and triggered MDSC expansion. On the other hand, ablation of the STAT3 gene using knockout mice or STAT3 blockade by tyrosine kinase inhibitor significantly reduced the number of tumor-associated MDSCs, which consequently elicited robust anti-tumor immune responses [6].

K-ras

K-ras is a member of a highly homologous group of approximately 21 kDa monomeric, membrane localized GTPases, which are involved in linking extracellular signals through membrane receptors to intracellular signals. The Ras family of monomeric G proteins which are H-ras, N-ras and K-ras, act as molecular switches, where the Ras proteins cycle from a GDP bound "off" state to a GTP bound "on" state in response to activation of various receptors. Activated Ras targets a number of downstream effectors such as Raf kinase, phosphoinositide 3'-kinase (PI3-K) and RalGEFs, which produce pleiotropic cellular effects including signaling in cell growth and survival of Ras in oncogenesis. Several K-ras point mutations are found to be constitutively activated with a high frequency in a variety of human tumors [7].

Of the three different Ras proteins which consist of H-, N- and K-ras, two alternatively spliced forms of K-ras exist, which are 4A and 4B. These alternative forms result in different c-terminal residues, which are important for post-translational modification. In total, the Ras superfamily consists of over 150 small GTPases and the *ras* genes share a potent ability to transform cells that are analogous of the Harvey and Kirsten sarcoma viruses for H- and K-ras and an oncogene N-ras, which has been isolated from neuroblastoma [7].

Activated Ras pathway is complex and Ras signaling is initiated by a wide range of stimuli. Ras activation begins with the stimulation of upstream receptors including receptor tyrosine kinases, integrins, serpentine receptors, heterotrimeric G-proteins and cytokine receptors. A well-known pathway of Ras stimulation is *via* a receptor tyrosine kinase such as EGF receptor. Once a ligand binds to EGF receptor, it induces oligomerization of the receptor, a process that results in juxtaposition of the cytoplasmic, catalytic domains in a manner that allows activation of the kinase activity and trans-phosphorylation. Adaptor proteins such as Grb2, then recognizes sequence homology 2 (SH2) domains followed by recruiting guanine nucleotide exchange factors (GEFs) such as SOS-1 or CDC25 to the cell membrane. The GEF is capable of interacting with Ras proteins at the cell membrane to promote conformational change and exchange GDP for GTP. Subcellular localization of GEFs is thought to play a key event in Ras activation. This was observed from SOS-1 or CDC25, which constitutively targeted to the cell membrane and enhanced the ability to transform NIH 3T3 cells. These exchanges also indicated that RAS regulates SOS activity involving bidirectional pathways. Ras activation is terminated upon hydrolysis of the GTP to GDP, although Ras proteins have intrinsically low GTPase activity. GTPase activity is stimulated by GAPs such as NF1-GAP/neurofibromin and inactivated by p120-GAP, thereby preventing prolonged Ras stimulated signaling. It needs to be mentioned that oncogenic transformation of *ras* mutation abolishes the interaction of GAPs and Ras. Normally, Ras signaling is transient because of the intrinsic GTPase activity and the action of GAPs. However, prolonged or constitutive Ras signaling as a result of *ras* mutation leads to NF-1 dysfunction or Ras overexpression and induces Ras mediated oncogenesis. In fact, K-ras mutation has been reported in a large number of solid tumors [7].

Not only in solid tumor, Ras was found to be deregulated also in leukemia. The frequency of mutation varies between different forms of leukemia with highest mutation rate is found in MDS and AML, which is approximately 30%. Loss of NF1 that we mentioned previously also correlated with the upregulation of Ras activity. Neurofibromatosis patients with loss of one wild-type NF1 allele are more likely to develop myeloid leukemia, especially juvenile chronic myeloid leukemia (JCML) [8]. In chronic myelomonocytic leukemia (CMML), PDGF receptor (PDGF-R) is affected by translocation t(5;12), which was found in a subset of CMML patients. Furthermore, wild-type Ras can be permanently activated through the BCR-ABL fusion, which is the result of the t(9;22) translocation and is also found in a subset of chronic myeloid leukemia (CML) patients. BCR-ABL activates Ras through permanent activation of Sos1. Bcl-2, which is a pro-survival protein of the Bcl-2 family of proteins, is induced by Ras activation which prevents apoptosis in hematopoietic cells, resulting in tumor growth [8].

Ras signaling is complex and involves many steps at which targeted therapies are designed to interfere with Ras signaling. Ras activation by tyrosine kinase and other receptors including EGFR, VEGFR, Her-2 and bcr-abl are potential targets for drug development against Ras. A successful cancer therapy designed to target Ras dysregulation should be orally active, have minimal systemic toxicity, and be a potential inhibitor of Ras activity. Till now, this type of agents are still unavailable. However, few of the targets that are under development are : (i) inhibitors of ras protein expression-(a) antisense oligonucleotides and (b) RNA interference; (ii) inhibitors of K-ras processing-(a) farnesyltransferase inhibitors, (b) combination of farnesyltransferase/geranyltrasferase inhibitors, (c) other Ras processing targets; (iii) targeting mutant K-ras protein-(a) immunological approaches, (b) mutant K-ras peptide inhibitors; (iv) targeting Ras effectors-(a) Raf kinase inhibitors, (b) MEK inhibitors, and (c) mTOR inhibitors [7]

MYC

The *myc*-family of genes include c-*myc*, L-*myc* and N-*myc*. These are proto-oncogenes and are activated in a variety of neoplasms. MYC was first discovered as an etiologic agent of retrovirally mediated tumorigenesis. MYC is over-expressed and/or activated in more than half of human cancers as a result of activation of both oncogenic and epigenetic events [9, 10].

MYC largely functions as a transcription factor that coordinates many biological processes. However, *Myc* activation can be a hallmark of cancer which is evident from autonomus proliferation and growth, continuous DNA replication, increased protein synthesis, global changes in cellular metabolism, activation of the angiogenic switch, suppression of the response to autocrine and paracrine regulatory programs and resistance to host immune system [9, 10].

MYC inactivation elicits oncogene addiction, *i.e.*, targeted inactivation of a single gene can induce dramatic tumor regression. Multiple mechanisms have been elucidated, which differ from tumor type. MYC inactivation in lymphoma induces proliferative arrest, differentiation, senescence and widespread apoptosis. In this case, MYC reactivation does not restore tumorigenesis. In liver adenocarcinoma, MYC inactivation induces proliferative arrest, differentiation, senescence and apoptosis. However, MYC reactivation can result in restoration of the tumor. Since MYC acts as a transcription factor, MYC has yet to be successfully therapeutically targeted for the treatment of cancer [9, 10].

However, recent research showed that oncogene addiction is highly dependent on the host immune cells. CD4+ helper T cells are shown to be essential to the mechanism by which MYC or BCR-ABL inactivation elicits "oncogene withdrawal" [11].

p53

p53 is another transcription factor which plays a tumor suppressor role by activating many genes involved in apoptosis and cell cycle arrest or senescence. P53 is also called "checkpoint" protein as it arrests cell cycle progression in the event of DNA damage, enabling DNA to be repaired. However, if the damage is excessive, p53 directs the cell towards apoptosis or programmed cell death (PCD). P53 is often mutated or inactivated in cancer, particularly Mdm2, which is a key p53-specific ubiquitin ligase. However, mutation in ARF, which controls the stability of Mdm2, also inactivates the p53 response [10].

Mutation in p53 or its regulatory proteins lacked response to chemotherapy. In acute lymphoblastic leukemia (ALL), the presence of wild type p53 correlated with a good response to therapy. However, the presence of functional or wild-type p53 showed different responses to radiation therapy [10].

Given the broad diversity in p53 controls and functions, p53 is reported to be associated with inflammation . P53 is upregulated at sites of inflammation. DNA damage that triggers p53 responses helps orchestrate clearance of damaged cells *via* the innate immune system. P53 dependent tumor regression was found to be related to tumor cell senescence program. P53 is also involved in the generation of immune cells. p53 acts as a modulator in stem cell appearance, which is reported from p53 in limiting expansion of hematopoietic stem cells (HSC) [12].

As p53 is a transcription factor, it can modulate the expression of several genes encoding enzymes involved in the production or elimination of reactive oxygen species ROS/NOS, upregulation of the antioxidant glutathione peroxidase (GPX1), aldehyde dehydrogenase 4 (ALDH1) and cyclooxygenase 2 (COX2). P53 is also able to repress directly or indirectly the expression of chemokines, which was observed from the loss of p53, leading to overexpression of proinflammatory chemokines such as CXCL2, -3, -5 and -8, CCL20, CCL28 and CXR4 in breast, ovarian and lung cancer cells. Conversely, chemokines can also influence p53 activities. The macrophage migration inhibitory factor (MIF), which is a product of activated macrophages, sustains macrophage survival and pro-inflammatory function by inhibiting p53 [12].

At present, nearly 30 immune-related genes (including miRNAs) targeted by p53 have been revealed. However, further studies are being conducted using high throughput sequencing (*e.g.*, chromatin immune-precipitation -ChIP-seq) and expression assays, which will elucidate p53 binding sites and this will help to identify candidate p53 target genes [8].

SIGNALING PATHWAYS ASSOCIATED WITH CANCER DEVELOPMENT

Apoptosis Pathway

Apoptosis is a programmed cell death (PCD) mechanism and is the most expected pathway to be activated in response to the different treatment modalities such as chemotherapy and radiotherapy to kill cancer cells. T cells and NK cells use death receptor and the granule exocytosis pathway. In the death receptor pathway, lymphocytes display the death ligand CD95L on the cell surface, which triggers apoptosis *via* the death receptor CD95 on the target cell. NK cells also use the death ligand TRAIL (tumor necrosis factor-TNF-related apoptosis-inducing ligand), which triggers apoptosis *via* the death receptors TRAIL-R1 or TRAIL-R2. These death receptors are members of the TNF receptor superfamily that comprises of an intracellular domain, the death domain. Cell killing mechanism by lymphocytes also depends on the induction of the apoptosis pathways. Lymphocytes induced apoptosis can be granzyme-perforin mediated killing and death ligand mediated killing. The former is performed by CD8+ CTL (CD4+ CTL) and NK cells and ADCC. The latter is mediated by TRAIL, FasL, TNF, CD4+ T cells, monocytes and dendritic cells [13].

Apoptosis can be induced by two pathways: intrinsic pathway of apoptosis and the extrinsic pathway of apoptosis. In both pathways, caspases, which are peptide molecules with specificity for tetra-peptide motifs-containing aspartate, play sequentially to kill the damaged or cancer cells. These proteins are synthesized as inactive proenzymes and upon proteolytic cleavage are activated. The caspase proteins are further divided into initiator caspases and effector caspases. The initiator caspases include caspase 8 and caspase 9 and these contain large pro-domains. Initiator caspases are able to self-activate in addition to activating the effector caspases which are caspase 3 or 7 [13].

The extrinsic pathway of apoptosis involves death receptors that are members of the tumor necrosis factor (TNF) receptor superfamily. These death receptors are further divided into subfamilies with varying intracellular death domains. Some of the death receptors include: CD95 (APO-1/Fas), TRAIL (TNF-related apoptosis-inducing ligand)-R1, TRAIL-R2, TNF-R1, DR3 and DR6. The extrinsic pathway is activated by death receptors at the cell surface. Once a ligand binds with the receptor, recruitment of intracellular adaptor proteins (*e.g.* FADD) and pro-caspases (*e.g.*, caspase 8 or 10) is undertaken. The receptor, adaptor protein and pro-caspase, altogether form the death-inducing complex (DISC). Once the DISC is formed, the caspases self-process and activate effector caspase. Pro-caspase 8 then undergoes autocatalysis and turns into the active form caspase 8. Activated caspase 8 then activates effector caspases, such as caspase 3, which executes the final stages of apoptosis and leads to apoptotic changes, such as chromatin condensation and blebbing [13].

Extrinsic pathway can be linked to the intrinsic pathway of apoptosis through cleavage of Bid. Activated caspase 8 cleaves Bid into t-Bid, which translocates to the mitochondria and activates the intrinsic pathway of apoptosis [13].

On the other hand, the intrinsic pathway of apoptosis, also known as the mitochondrial pathway of apoptosis, is regulated by a Bcl2 family of proteins. The Bcl2 family of protein consists of anti-apoptotic protein and pro-apoptotic protein. The anti-apoptotic proteins are: Bcl2, Bcl-xL, Mcl-1, Bcl-W and A1. The pro-apoptotic proteins are Bax and Bak. Pro-apoptotic BH3 damages sensor proteins such as Bid, Bik, Bim, Bmf, Noxa, Puma, Bad and Hrk [13].

In addition to the Bcl2 group of proteins, other regulators of the apoptosis pathways include phosphatidylinositol 3-kinase (PI3K-Akt, NF-κB and Ras-Ra--MEK-ERK pathways. In normal cells, the survival and apoptotic signaling pathways contribute to a complex signaling network that regulates proper cell growth. However, many of these genes or proteins are mutated in cancer cells and contribute to tumor growth. For example, the Bcl2 family proteins play anti-apoptotic role in leukemia and solid tumor development. An inhibitor, ABT737, binds to the surfaces of the Bcl2 family of protein and blocks the anti-apoptotic activity of Mcl-1 [14].

While the molecules associated with apoptosis signal transduction pathways have been studied in many types of cancers involving the immune system, only a few are known to be associated with immune escape mechanisms. Studies in mice xenograft model showed that neutralization of TRAIL promoted tumor development in mice. Mutation in CD95L developed B cell malignancies. Studies showed that overexpression of apoptotic molecules, FLIP, interferes with apoptosis induction at the level of death receptors, *i.e.*, by extrinsic pathway of apoptosis, and does not prevent the perforin/granzyme mediated apoptosis. Tumors with high expression of FLIP showed escape from T-cell mediated immunity *in vivo* despite the presence of the perforin/granzyme pathway. FLIP overexpression prevents rejection of tumors by perforin-deficient NK cells. High levels of FLIP were observed in human melanomas and Epstein-Barr virus-positive Burkitt's lymphoma cell lines. In the latter case, increased ratio of FLIP to caspase-8 correlated with resistance to CD95-mediated apoptosis. A number of tumorogenic viruses such as Kaposi sarcoma-associated herpesvirus (KSHV) encode viral analogs of FLIP (v-FLIPs). KSHV-FLIP promotes tumor establishment and growth in immunocompetent mice by preventing death-receptor induced apoptosis mediated my T cells, which contribute to immune escape of v-FLIP-encoding viruses [14].

Other anti-apoptotic proteins are also involved in apoptosis resistance of tumors. Enhanced Bcl-2 expression is found in follicular B-cell lymphoma (Bcl) with the chromosomal translocation t(14;18), which is known to couple the Bcl-2 gene to the immunoglobulin heavy chain locus. Bcl-2 also contributes to tumorigenesis in cooperation with the oncogenes c-Myc or promyelocytic leukemia retinoic acid receptor alpha. Bcl-2expression also correlates with different grades of human tumors. Bcl-2 expression confers resistance to CD95L and other apoptosis stimuli. Its high level of expression is associated with poor disease-free survival. Furthermore, tumor associated viruses such as Epstein-Barr virus and human KSHV encode proteins that are homologs of Bcl-2, leading to tumorigenesis [13, 15].

Autophagy Pathway

Autophagy is a lysosomal degradation pathway which once induced, leads to the formation of double-membrane autophagic vesicles (AV) or autophagosomes followed by engulfment of cytoplasmic contents along with damaged organelles, protein aggregates and bacteria. Autophagy is a highly conserved process among eukaryotic cells. It includes a number of steps for AV production and turnover such as initiation, nucleation, and maturation of AVs and fusion and degradation of AV contents in lysosomes [16].

There are three morphologically distinct forms of autophagy, macroautophagy, microautophagy and chaperone-mediated autophagy. Of these, macroautopahgy is distinguished by the double membrane vesicle mentioned above and the source of the membrane is thought to be originated from endoplasmic reticulum (ER) membrane. The other two forms of autophagy are characterized by direct membrane invagination of damaged proteins and a specific process involving translocation of the targeted proteins across the lysosomal membrane. Since macroautophagy is associated with different types of cancer, we will elaborate on the modu017ors of this pathway in the context of signal transduction and cancer progression [16].

The macroautopahgy is regulated by a number of modulators such as mammalian target of rapamycin (mTOR), phosphatidylinositol 3-kinase (PI3K), *etc.* Of these, mTOR is a serine threonine kinase and is known to regulate cell growth, protein synthesis, metabolism and cell death. mTOR is an inhibitor of the autophagy pathway. It regulates metabolic stress signals to drive cellular growth and development in the presence of nutrient abundance. Upstream of mTOR is the PI3K pathway, which most notably regulates cellular proliferation. Class I PI3K is a signal transducer which receives signals from upstream growth factors and facilitates phosphorylation of Akt. Akt, also known as protein kinase B, by 3-phosphoinositide-dependent kinase 1 (PDK1), is associated with cell survival pathway. Once Akt is phosphorylated, mTOR is activated and autophagy is inhibited [16].

Downstream of mTOR is the ULK (unc-51-like kinase) complex composed of Atg13 (autophagy related gene 13), ULK1/2, and family interacting protein (FIP200), all of which are required for the initiation of autophagosome formation. Under normal metabolic conditions, mTOR phosphorylates Atg13, disrupting binding of ULK1, ULK2 and FIP200. During energy deprivation, AMP activated protein kinase (AMPK) is activated, leading to inhibition of mTOR and consequent activation of the ULK kinase complex and initiation of auto-phagosome formation [16].

Signals from ULK1 kinase complex are critical for progression of autophagy as these signals initiate vacuolar sorting protein 34 (Vps34), which then binds with beclin-1, a promoter of autophagy, to form the beclin-1 complex. This complex then recruits and facilitates as a binding site for other Atg proteins to bind and drive the early steps of autophagosome formation. The function of beclin-1 can be suppressed or activated through different binding partners such as Bcl-2 (B-cell lymphoma2), which is a cell death regulating protein, and activated by the tumor-suppressing gene UVRAG (UV radiation resistance-associated gene) [16].

Another regulator of autophagy is p53, which is a tumor suppressor gene. Its regulatory function is location-dependent. Nuclear p53 induces autophagy by activating target genes DRAM (damaged-regulated autophagy modulator). On the other hand, cytoplasmic p53 inhibits autophagy pathway in a cell-cycle dependent manner [16].

Autophagy has been found to be an important regulator of the innate immune response. In breast cancer, hypoxia impairs breast cancer cell susceptibility to NK-mediated lysis *in vitro via* the activation of autophagy. Inhibition of autophagy by targeting beclin1 (BECN1) restored granzyme B levels in hypoxic cells and induced tumor regression *in vivo* by facilitating NK-mediated tumor cell killing [17].

Autophagy is also associated with the progression of other cancers such as colon cancer or solid tumors. A number of autophagy pathway inhibitors are at clinical trial stage [18].

CONCLUSION

The chromosomal anomalies in the cancer cell include polyploidy, aneuploidy and gross chromosomal rearrangements by translocations. Other changes include mutations in proto-oncogenes that convert these genes into dominant oncogenes and mutation in tumor suppressor genes. Furthermore, epigenetic changes also occur and involve loss of DNA methylation and alteration in histone acetylation. These genetic and epigenetic changes lead to cell immortalization, transform cancer cells into metastatic cancer cells with the continuation of genomic instability and the consequent changes as long as the cancer cell is alive. Signal transduction pathways play important role in establishing crosstalk between external stimuli and the internal ligand receptors. Cancer cells have unstable genome. Identification of the specific signaling proteins involved in cancer progression can be an important strategy to develop target based therapies. A number of inhibitors are currently under clinical trials to be used as anticancer drugs. However, tumor cells do not depend on single signaling molecules. They are constantly evolving entities and are heterogeneous in their cellular makeup. Moreover, it is not known whether these targeted therapies can be used as combination drugs with immunotherapy.

CONFLICT OF INTEREST

The author confirms that author has no conflict of interest to declare for this publication.

ACKNOWLEDGEMENTS

Decleared none.

REFERENCES

[1]   Wu W, Hu C. Microenvironment triggers EMT, migration and invasion of primary tumor *via* multiple signal pathways. In: Wu W-S, Hu C-T, Eds. Signal Transduct Cancer Metastasis. Dordrecht: Springer Netherlands 2010; pp. 9-24.
[http://dx.doi.org/10.1007/978-90-481-9522-0_2]

[2]   Chosdol K, Bhagat M, Dikshit B, *et al.* Nuclear factors linking cancer and infl ammation. In: Kumar R, Ed. Nucl signal pathways target transcr cancer springer science+ business media. New York: LLC Landes Bioscience 2014; pp. 121-54.
[http://dx.doi.org/10.1007/978-1-4614-8039-6_6]

[3]   Teng Y, Ross JL, Cowell JK. The involvement of JAK-STAT3 in cell motility, invasion, and metastasis. JAK-STAT 2014; 3(1): e28086.
[http://dx.doi.org/10.4161/jkst.28086] [PMID: 24778926]

[4]   Grivennikov SI, Greten FR, Karin M. Immunity, inflammation, and cancer. Cell 2010; 140(6): 883-99.
[http://dx.doi.org/10.1016/j.cell.2010.01.025] [PMID: 20303878]

[5]   Shuai K, Liu B. Regulation of JAK-STAT signalling in the immune system. Nat Rev Immunol 2003; 3(11): 900-11.
[http://dx.doi.org/10.1038/nri1226] [PMID: 14668806]

[6]   Lee H, Pal SK, Reckamp K, *et al.* STAT3 : A Target to Enhance Antitumor Immune Response. Cancer Immunother tumor Immunol 2011; 41-59.

[7]   Friday BB. Adjei A a (2005) K-ras as a target for cancer therapy. Biochim Biophys Acta 2005; 1756: 127-44.
[http://dx.doi.org/10.1016/j.bbcan.2005.08.001]

[8]   Weijzen S, Velders MP, Kast WM. Modulation of the immune response and tumor growth by activated Ras. Leukemia 1999; 13(4): 502-13.
[http://dx.doi.org/10.1038/sj.leu.2401367] [PMID: 10214854]

[9]   Gabay M. MYC Activation Is a Hallmark of Cancer Initiation.pdf. Cold Spring Harb Perspect Med 2014; 1-13.

[10]   Levitzki A, Klein S. Signal transduction therapy of cancer. Mol Aspects Med 2010; 31(4): 287-329.
       [http://dx.doi.org/10.1016/j.mam.2010.04.001] [PMID: 20451549]

[11]   Casey SC, Li Y, Fan AC, Felsher DW. Oncogene withdrawal engages the immune system to induce sustained cancer regression. J Immunother Cancer 2014; 2: 24.
       [http://dx.doi.org/10.1186/2051-1426-2-24] [PMID: 25089198]

[12]   Lowe J, Shatz M, Resnick M, Menendez D. Modulation of immune responses by the tumor suppressor p53. Biodiscovery 2013; 2: 1-13.

[13]   Wu W, Wu J. Overview of signal transduction in tumor metastasis. In: Wu W, Ed. Signal Transduct cancer metastasis. China 2010; pp. 1-8.
       [http://dx.doi.org/10.1007/978-90-481-9522-0_1]

[14]   Zhang P, Zweidler-mckay PA. Signal Transduction in Cancer Metastasis 2010; 15: 157-74.
       [http://dx.doi.org/10.1007/978-90-481-9522-0_9]

[15]   Igney FH, Krammer PH. Immune escape of tumors : apoptosis resistance and tumor counterattack. J Leukoc Biol 2002; 71(6): 907-20.;

[16]   Duffy A, Le J, Sausville E, Emadi A. Autophagy modulation: a target for cancer treatment development. Cancer Chemother Pharmacol 2015; 75(3): 439-47.
       [http://dx.doi.org/10.1007/s00280-014-2637-z] [PMID: 25422156]

[17]   Baginska J, Viry E, Berchem G, *et al.* Granzyme B degradation by autophagy decreases tumor cell susceptibility to natural killer-mediated lysis under hypoxia. Proc Natl Acad Sci USA 2013; 110(43): 17450-5.
       [http://dx.doi.org/10.1073/pnas.1304790110] [PMID: 24101526]

[18]   Janji B, Viry E, Baginska J. Role of autophagy in cancer and tumor progression. Autohpagy-A double-edged sword_cell surviv or death. Croatia, EU: Intech 2013; pp. 189-216.
       [http://dx.doi.org/10.5772/55388]

CHAPTER 4

Cancer Immunotherapy

Abstract: Treatment of cancer does not depend on a single drug and the existing strategies are challenged by the the frequent development of drug resistance properties of cancer cells. Although chemotherapy drugs are still used as the first line of treatment modalities for cancer, immunotherapyis also used as a targeted treatment modality nowadays. However, major challenge with the treatment is that, patient recovery is very low. Therefore, combination therapies are being investigated and some of them are at the clinical stage with FDA approval. In this chapter, we will discuss currently available immunotherapy drugs and their synergistic effects in combination with chemotherapy drugs or two different immunotherapy drugs

Keywords: Checkpoint blockades Chemotherapy, Combination therapy, Immunotherapy, Monoclonal antibodies, Synergistic, Vaccines.

INTRODUCTION

Cancer is treated either locally or by applying drugs. The main difference between these two approaches is that, local treatments are performed by surgery and radiotherapy whereas drugs are used for systemic treatment. At present, four different categories of drugs are used to treat cancer. These include chemotherapy, hormonal therapy, targeted therapy and immunotherapy. Of these, chemotherapies involve a large group of cytotoxic drugs and they interfere with cell division and DNA synthesis. Hormonal therapies interfere with growth signaling through hormone receptors on cancer cells. Targeted therapies involve a group of antibodies and small molecule-kinase inhibitors that specifically target the growth signaling pathways in cancer cells. Immunotherapies induce or augment anti-cancer immune responses [1 - 3].

Of the different types of cancer drugs, the concept of immunotherapy dates back to the late nineteenth century during which tumor shrinkage was observed following administration of bacterial products in and around tumors. At that time, antibodies were recognized as "magic bullets" for cancer therapy. Since then many observations were documented including spontaneous remissions of cancer, higher incidences of cancer in immuno-suppressed patients and identification of tumor specific antigens and lymphocytes. In addition, considerable knowledge has been obtained by investigating the components that either induce or enhance the anti-tumor immune responses. Agents and products that enhance the immune system include non-specific inflammatory inducers such as bacterial lipo-polysaccharides (LPS), tumor associated antigens (TAA), cytokines and antibodies (Abs). Components of the immune system that are used as cancer therapy include cytokines, immune cells and monoclonal antibodies (mAbs) [1, 2].

Despite its discovery almost a century ago, several factors hampered the development of cancer immunotherapy. Two major obstacles are: (i) the presence of the immunosuppressive cells of the tumor microenvironment; and (ii) challenges of designing immunotherapy trials [1, 2].

We already know from the previous chapters that tumor microenvironment is a highly dynamic system and it is able to avoid and escape the immune system (ref: cancer immunotherapy- revisited). Thus, tumor evolution proceeds through induced immunosuppression and adaptation to immune recognition by altering the expression of surface markers. The presence of tumor associated macrophages (TAM), T regulatory cells (Treg) and myeloid derived suppressor cells (MDSCs) forms immune suppressive network in tumor microenvironment. The presence of these diverse suppressed populations in tumor environment is an obstacle in increasing effective immune response for tumor elimination [1, 2, 5, 6].

Obstacles associated with designing the clinical trials include difficulty to define the optimal dose and schedule for immunotherapies. Compared to classical chemotherapeutic agents, there is insufficient correlation between the maximal tolerated dose and the maximal effective dose. Another problem associated with immunotherapies is that the classical volumetric response criteria are inadequate for evaluating the efficacy of immunotherapy. Immunotherapy is favorable for testing the drug in a low volume and or microscopic stage but less effective in patients with a large tumor burden [1, 2]. Another difficulty with immuno-therapies that hampered the clinical development of many immunotherapies is lack of patentability and lack of funding by pharmaceuticals [7]. Despite these difficulties and drawbacks, some recent pre-clinical and clinical findings have given a great boost to immunotherapy and several of them also received approval from the US Food and Drug Administration (FDA) [7].

Not only immunotherapy drugs, but other treatment modalities of cancer (*e.g.*, chemotherapy drugs) also induce immune response. Therefore, combination treatment modalities can be used to design synergistic treatment modalities. In this chapter, we will discuss different types of immunotherapy drugs and their effect on the immune systems, clinical phases and trials and effects of the combination therapies on the immune system.

CHEMOTHERAPY DRUGS AND THE IMMUNE SYSTEM

Chemotherapy drugs are used as the first line of treatment modalities for different types of cancer. Chemotherapies are used as drug or medicine and differ from other treatment strategies such as surgery and radiotherapy as these are localized treatments and chemotherapy is a systemic treatment. Currently, more than 100 different types of chemotherapies are known and these are broadly classified based on their chemical structure [3, 8]. Most of the chemotherapy drugs are cytotoxic to the cancer cells. Cell death following treatment with chemotherapy may or may not induce immunogenic response. The non- immunogenic death can be either apoptotic death or non-apoptotic death. The apoptotic death in response to anticancer drug is mediated by death-receptor-dependent and independent pathways. Anticancer drugs such as 5-FU increases the expression of death receptors FAS, tumor necrosis factor (TNF) and TNF related ligand receptors. Other anticancer drugs trigger apoptosis by inducing the release of cytochrome c from mitochondria. The non-apoptotic death includes necrosis and mitotic cell death and characterized by inhibition of cell cycle. However, the frequency of non-apoptotic death is less compared to apoptotic death [7, 9].

Chemotherapy drugs can induce immune response too. Immunogenic cell death induces maturation of dendritic cells (DC) followed by activation of relevant T cells [9]. However, some drugs can induce both pathways and this depends on the concentration of the drug used and the type of tumor cells. For example, 5-fuoruracil (5-FU) induces either the death receptor pathway or death receptor independent pathway in colorectal cancer cell lines *in vitro*. The induction of the pathways depends on the concentration of the chemotherapy drug and the type of tumor cells (either sensitive or resistant cell lines) [6, 13]. Other drugs such as cytarabine, mitoxantrone, etoposide and topotecan increase the number of apoptotic cells in leukemia and the degree of apoptosis correlates with clinical outcome for different tumor types [6].

Table 1. Major types of chemotherapies currently used to treat cancer [5, 11].

Type	Mechanism	Example	Side effects
Alkylating agents	Modification of nucleic acid functional groups.	Nitrogen mustard *e.g.* mechlorethamine, Nitrosoureas *e.g.* streptozocin, Alkyl sulfonates *e.g.* busulfan, Triazines *e.g.* dacarbazine (DTIC) and Ethylenimines *e.g.* thiotepa	Cytotoxicity may lead to hair loss, breathlessness, fatigue, eating challenges, memory and thinking dysfunction, nausea, neutropenia and pain. Recurrence Drug resistance
Antimetabolites	Nucleoside analogs, interfere with RNA and DNA synthesis.	5-fluorouracil (5-FU), 6-mercaptopurine (6-MP), Capecitabine, Floxuridine, Fludarabine, Gemcitabine, Hydroxyurea, Methotrexate, Pentostatin, Thioguanine	
Anti-tumor antibiotics (anthracyclines)	Interferes with DNA replication, inhibits RNA and DNA synthesis.	Doxorubicin, Actinomycin-D	Treatment related leukemia
Topoisomerase inhibitors	Inhibits DNA unwinding	Topotecan and irinotecan (CPT-11), etoposide (VP-16), teniposide	Increased risk of secondary cancer or relapses
Mitotic inhibtors (taxanes)	Disruption of microtubule formation and stops cell division	Paclitaxel, docetaxel, ixabepilone, vinblastine	Cause peripheral nerve damage
Platinum based	Cross links DNA, triggers apoptosis	Cisplatin, carboplatin, oxaliplatin	Kidney damage, nerve damage, nausea and vominitng, hearing loss, electrolyte disturbance, bone marrow suppression and haemolytic anemia.

A major problem with the chemotherapy dependent treatment strategies is that these drugs are cytotoxic for both normal and malignant cells and most of the drugs function in non-specific manner (Table **1**). Another worth mentioning disadvantage of the chemotherapy drugs is that cancer cells develop resistance against the chemotherapies, which causes relapses of the treatment of cancer. Mechanisms by which cancer cells develop chemo-resistance are: (i) decreased drug uptake; (ii) decreased drug activation; (iii) increased drug target; (iv) detoxification; (v) enhanced repair (vi) increased efflux; (vii) defective DNA repair; and (viii) mutation in tumor suppressor genes [10]. Despite the drawbacks, chemotherapy drugs are not only used as primary therapy but also as neo-adjuvant therapy and combination therapy [10]. The use depends on the stage of the disease. However, their use as adjuvants, neo-adjuvants and combination therapies is based on several factors such as: (i) selection of drug to be active in metastatic setting; (ii) the drug selected should have different mechanisms of action; (iii) the drugs should not have overlapping toxicities; (iv) all drugs should be given at full dose and at an optimal schedule; and (v) dosing intervals should be consistent and short [10].

Immuno-modulation of Chemotherapy Drugs

Chemotherapy drugs kill cancer cells either by apoptotic mechanism or by non-apoptotic mechanism. Apoptotic death occurs either by death receptor dependent pathway (also known as extrinsic pathway of apoptosis) or by death receptor independent pathway (also known as intrinsic pathway of apoptosis). Some anticancer drugs increase the expression of death receptors such as FAS, tumor-necrosis factor (TNF) receptors and TNF-related apoptosis inducing ligand receptors. On the other hand, some drugs do not alter the expression of death receptors and trigger apoptosis by inducing release of cytochrome *c* from mitochondria. However, some drugs can induce both pathways and this depends on the concentration of the drug used and the type of tumor cells. For example, 5-fuoruracil (5-FU) induces either the death receptor pathway or death receptor independent pathway in colorectal cancer cell lines *in vitro*. The induction of the pathways depends on the concentration of the chemotherapy drug and the type of tumor cells (either sensitive or resistant cell lines) [6, 13]. Other drugs such as cytarabine, mitoxantrone, etoposide and topotecan increase the number of apoptotic cells in leukemia and the degree of apoptosis correlates with clinical outcome for several different tumor types [6].

Bonotte and colleagues showed that some part of the apoptotic process generates immune reaction. For example, it was reported that immunogenic colon cancer cells are sensitive to apoptosis *in vitro* if these cells were starved with growth factors. The cells showed resistance to apoptosis if the anti-apoptotic protein BCL2 was overexpressed [6].

Some vaccine strategies, including cancer vaccines, rely on apoptosis for immunogenic response. Phosphatidyl serine (PS) is a membrane component and involved in cell signaling. PS becomes accessible to macrophages after non-apoptotic cell death during which the plasma membrane loses its integrity. PS functions as a down-regulator of immune response. It stimulates the production of a number of anti-inflammatory mediators such as transforming growth factor-β (TGF- β), prostanoids, and interleukin-10 (IL-10).transforming growth factor-β (TGF- β), prostanoids, and interleukin-10 (IL-10). In the absence of a signal, PS recognition suppresses the release of pro- inflammatory cytokines (*e.g.*, IL-12). This occurs through transcriptional repression of p35 IL-12 subunit, leading to loss of IL-12 production [6, 14].

In case of massive apoptosis, immune function is activated by heat shock proteins (HSPs). These proteins are induced by stressed apoptotic leukemic cells and increase the activation of DCs. Moreover, phagocytosis of apoptotic cells increases secretion of growth and survival factors such as vascular endothelial growth factor (VEGF). Uric acid, released from injured cells, plays important role as endogenous pro-inflammatory signal. These studies revealed that apoptosis is not induced by single response. Instead, these are induced by the amount of cellular stress and the pattern of regulatory cytokines [6].

On the other hand, non-apoptotic death includes necrosis, autophagy and mitotic catastrophe. Temozolomide, which is an alkylating agent and a chemotherapy drug, induces cell cycle arrest at G2/M phase of growth without inducing apoptosis. Necrosis death might induce DCs that act as potent APCs. These immune responses were observed in *in vitro* condition [6].

Majority of the chemotherapy drugs target rapidly dividing cells. As a result, this also affects the T cells that are present in the tumor microenvironment. Intensive chemotherapy causes lymphopenia, leading to decreased percentage of circulating T cells and blunt anti-tumor response. However, several researches showed that chemotherapies used at non-cytotoxic doses can induce the antitumor response. For example, drugs like paclitaxel, doxorubicin, mitomycin C and methotrexate induce antigen presentation in an autocrine IL-12 dependent manner. Dendritic cells treated with vinblastine induced CD8+ T cell responses. Treatment of myeloma cells with proteasome inhibitor bortezomib expresses heat shock protein HSP90 on the cell surface and gives "eat me" signals to DCs. 5-Fluorouracil (5-FU), CPT-11 and cisplatin (CIS) increased cancer cell death in SW480 colon cancer cell line by CTLs. Chemotherapies can also eliminate MDSC and Tregs, thus removing some of the immunosuppressive factors in cancer patients [4]. While these were observed only under non-cytotoxic doses, cancer patients treated with the conventional dose of chemotherapy did not show these responses as these depend on the type of cancer, stage of cancer and patient'scharacteristics. Therefore, the combined effect of immunotherapy and chemotherapy could be used to treat cancer patients.

Treatments involving combination therapy use chemotherapy as adjuvant therapy. However, modulation of the immune system depends on the type of cancer and the choice of the particular chemotherapy drug. A favorable immune response to tumor elimination and lyses involves generation of large numbers of interferon-γ (IFN γ) and TNFα-secreting CD8+ T cells that are specific to the tumor antigen. Six key steps play important rolein CD8+ mediated anti-tumor immunity. These include: (i) antigen threshold: requiring the presence of tumor antigen; (ii) antigen presentation: the antigen must reach antigen presenting cells (APCs) in the draining lymph node; (iii) T cell response: specific T cells must respond by proliferation; (iv) T cell trafficking: circulating T cells must enter the tumor; (v) target destruction: these T cells must overcome local immune-suppressive molecules to recognize and kill the targets; and (vi) generation of memory: memory T cells must be generated. Since immunotherapy can fail at any of these steps, key issues in pairing chemotherapy with immunotherapy will be to identify molecular flags associated with different forms of cell death and how they are contextually interpreted [6].

Chemotherapy drugs can augment the effect of immunotherapy drugs in a number of ways, including: (i) increase antigen threshold by delivery of a broad range of different tumor antigens; (ii) enhance antigen presentation through increased antigen cross presentation, partial activation of DCs, priming of APCs for CD40 signal and killing subsets of APC; (iii) induction of T-cell response through no tolerance induction by apoptotic tumor and lymphopenia related proliferation increases tumor specific T-cell response; (iv)T-cell traffic: increased T-cell accumulation within tumor; (v) target destruction: increased local tumor antigen cross-presentation to permit CD8 restimulation, tumor debulking to lessen systemic suppression, less chance for escape variants, *etc.*; (vi) generation of memory: promotion of long-term antigen independent memory; (vii) external regulation by external delivery of exogenous antigen, increased CD4 help (*e.g.*, delivery of CD40 signals), reduction in function of negative regulatory cells and induction of homeostatic proliferation; (viii) elimination of cells with immuno-suppressive activity such as the myeloid derived suppressor cells (MDSCs) and regulatory T cells (Treg); (ix) non-specific activation of antigen presenting cells; (x) disruption of tumor stroma that results in improved penetration of CTLs into the tumor site; (xi) decreased local suppressive activity of tumor cells *via* mechanisms involving program death ligands (PDL), indoleamine 2,3-dioxygenase (IDO), or immunosuppressive cytokines; (xii) increased permeability of tumor cells to CTL derived granzymes; (xiii) increased expression of tumor associated antigens by tumor cells that could make them more available for targeting by CTLs; (xiv) up-regulation of Fas and other death receptors on tumor cells, or FasL on CTLs;and (xv) synergistic effect on caspase 3 activation between chemotherapeutics, granzymes and Fas [1, 6, 15].

IMMUNOTHERAPY AND THE IMMUNE SYSTEM

Cancer immunotherapy was first introduced by Coley in 1890. However, the clinical benefit of cancer immunotherapy was initially less and its resurgence as a treatment option for cancer occurred in 1997. Until now, FDA has approved 12 monoclonal antibodies. Ideally, immunotherapy is expected to function and contribute to an effective immune response by fulfiling several key characteristics. These are specificity, trafficking, adaptability and durability or memory [15].

According to the National Cancer Institute, immunotherapies are those that boost or restore the ability of the immune system to fight against diseases such as cancer, infections or other types of diseases [15]. Currently, immunotherapies used for cancer are classified in a number of ways.

Immunotherapy can be classified based on how they engage the immune system (*e.g.*, active therapy or passive therapy). Passive immunotherapies include monoclonal antibody and cytokine and they do not generate immunologic memory. Instead, these enhance pre-existing immune response. Passive immunotherapies are considered short lived and require constant administration to elicit an effect. On the contrary, active immunotherapy stimulates host immune system in such a way that it generates immunologic memory and durable effect even after the treatment has stopped [15], depending on howit engages the patient's immune system (*e.g.*, active therapy or passive therapy). Passive immunotherapy is based on the use of an agent or cell type which is administered to the patient to initiate an anti-tumor effect. Immune therapies using monoclonal antibody and cytokine are passive immunotherapies. In general, passive therapies do not generate immunologic memory, but enhance pre-existing immune response. These are considered as short lived, and consequently may require chronic administration to elicit an effect. In contrast, active immunotherapy stimulates the host immune system, and based on how these are generated, active immunotherapy can generate immunologic memory and durable effect even after the treatment has stopped [15].

Immunotherapy can be further classified as specific therapy and non-specific therapy. Each of these has distinct mechanisms of actions. Both of these are designed to induce the immune function in some manner [15]. Cytokines and non-specific adjuvants produce a wide range of anti- tumor effect and therefore these are considered as non-specific immunotherapy. Monoclonal antibodies and cancer vaccines produce specific immune response to a target antigen and therefore considered as specific immunotherapy [15]. Checkpoint inhibitors have characteristics of both active immunotherapy and passive immunotherapy. Active immunotherapies are also used in personalized medicine [15].

NON-SPECIFIC CANCER IMMUNOTHERAPY AND ADJUVANTS

Non-specific immunotherapy stimulates the immune system in a more general way as compared to the targeted therapies. Several natural and synthetic products can elicit immune response and non-specific inflammation that can affect cancer cells. Various bacterial polysaccharides and glycoproteins can induce the immune system. In addition, several immune modulators including cytokines and interferons and a variety of thymus extracts can induce the immune system [3].

Bacillus Calmette-Guerin (BCG)

BCG was developed as an attenuated strain of *Mycobacterium bovis* in 1906 to be used as vaccine to prevent tuberculosis. In 1970, it was evaluated as a treatment for cancer *via* intra-lesional injection to treat melanoma. BCG was also used as subcutaneous or intradermal non-specific immune stimulator for various malignancies. BCG (Tice®) was granted FDA approval in 1990 for the intravesical treatment of superficial bladder cancer. It is still considered as first line of treatment for *in situ* bladder cancer. BCG is also used as an adjuvant for various types of cancer vaccines, although it failed to show benefit as an adjuvant for breast cancer or melanoma [3]. The precise mechanism by which BCG exerts its anti-tumor effect is still unknown. Research showed that after instillation of BCG, the bacteria is internalized by the bladder epithelium and the resulting mycobacteria glycoprotein complexes induce an inflammatory response involving cellular infiltration and the local release of cytotoxic cytokines [3].

Levamisole

Levamisole Levamisole (Ergamasol®) belongs to synthetic phenylimidazothiazole oral antihelminthic group. It received FDA approval in 1990 as an adjuvant for the treatment of colon cancer. Combination of 5FU and levamisole reduced the risk or recurrence and death of colon cancer patients with either locally invasive or metastatic to regional lymph nodes cancer. The combination was more effective for patients with lymph node metastases. Although this combination was standard therapy for the treatment of stage III colon cancer during 1990-1997, the randomized trials failed to show benefit for this combination [3].

Cytokines

Cytokines are protein molecules that are secreted by cells and play role in cell signaling and immune response. Their anticancer effects are believed to be mediated by their effects on immune cells. Numerous cytokines are used to treat cancer, including hematopoietic colony- stimulating factors (CSFs), interferons (IFNs), interleukins (ILs), tumor necrosis factors (TNF), and a number of protein ligands. A number of cytokines have received FDA approval. These include erythropoietin (EPO), granulocytes CSF (G- CSF), and granulocyte-macrophage CSF (GM-CSF), IFN-α and IL-2 [2].

Interferon-α

Interferons (IFNs) are a large family of immune regulatory proteins. They are characterized as α, β, γ and ω. IFN- α was the first biological or immunotherapy that received regulatory approval in 1986 as an anticancer agent. It was originally isolated from leukocytes and the gene for IFN- α was cloned and the product was produced by recombinant DNA techniques. While IFN- α interferes with viral replication, various IFNs also have wide range of immune- stimulating effects including direct cytostatic effects on tumor cells. Two recombinant DNA products that were extensively studied and eventually approved for widespread use are interferon- α2a (Intron A®) and interferon- α2b (Roferon®) [2]. IFN- α has been approved to be used in virtually every malignancy such as hairy-cell leukemia, AIDS-related Kaposi's sarcoma, follicular lymphoma, chronic myeloid leukemia (CML) and metastatic melanoma. Disadvantage of IFN- α is that, it has a broad spectrum of toxicity that is dose related and leads to lethal hepatic toxicity [2].

Interleukins

Interleukins (ILs) take part in signal transduction between white blood cells. At least 35 ILs have been reported to play anti-cancer role. Of these, IL-2 helps immune system cells to grow and divide at a faster rate compared to other interleukins. A modified IL-2 (Proleukin®) has been approved to treat advanced kidney cancer and metastatic melanoma. IL-2 was originally isolated as secretion component from media that had antigen-activated helper T-cells. IL-2 gene was cloned by recombinant DNA technique for large scale production. It does not have any direct anti-tumor effect but induces cytotoxic natural-killer (NK) and T-lymphocytes [2].

Granulocyte-Macrophage Colony-Stimulating Factor (GM-CSF)

GM-CSF is a cytokine which plays important role in differentiation of myeloid cells. It is one of the hematopoietic stimulating factors and has been approved for clinical use. Its effect on monocytes, macrophages and dendritic cells is of great significance for immunotherapy. It has been used as an adjuvant with vaccines where GN-CSF is either co-administered or has been genetically modified for the vaccine product [2].

MONOCLONAL ANTIBODIES

Our immune system produces large number of antibodies once a foreign substance attacks the body. Antibodies are protein molecules that are produced in response to a specific protein of the foreign substance called antigen. Inside the body, plasma cells that originate from B cells produce antibodies. Antibodies circulate in the blood until they recognize an antigen and attach to it. We know that our immune system recognizes only foreign antigens and gives rise to a particular antibody, avoiding any 'self' antigen. Clonal selection helps the immune system to respond to a particular antigen. Once an antibody attaches to an antigen, it generates signals to the other cells of the immune system to destroy the cells that present the antigen (APCs) [6, 16, 19].

The mechanisms by which mAbs kill tumor cells can be direct cell killing, immune-mediated tumor cell killing and vascular and stromal ablation. Direct tumor cell killing can be through cell surface receptor agonist activity leading to apoptosis; through receptor blockade by inhibiting signaling, reducing proliferation and induce apoptosis; and through cell surface enzyme neutralization leading to signaling abrogation or by delivery of a drug, radiation, or cytotoxic agent by conjugated antibody (Fig. **1**) [6, 16, 20].

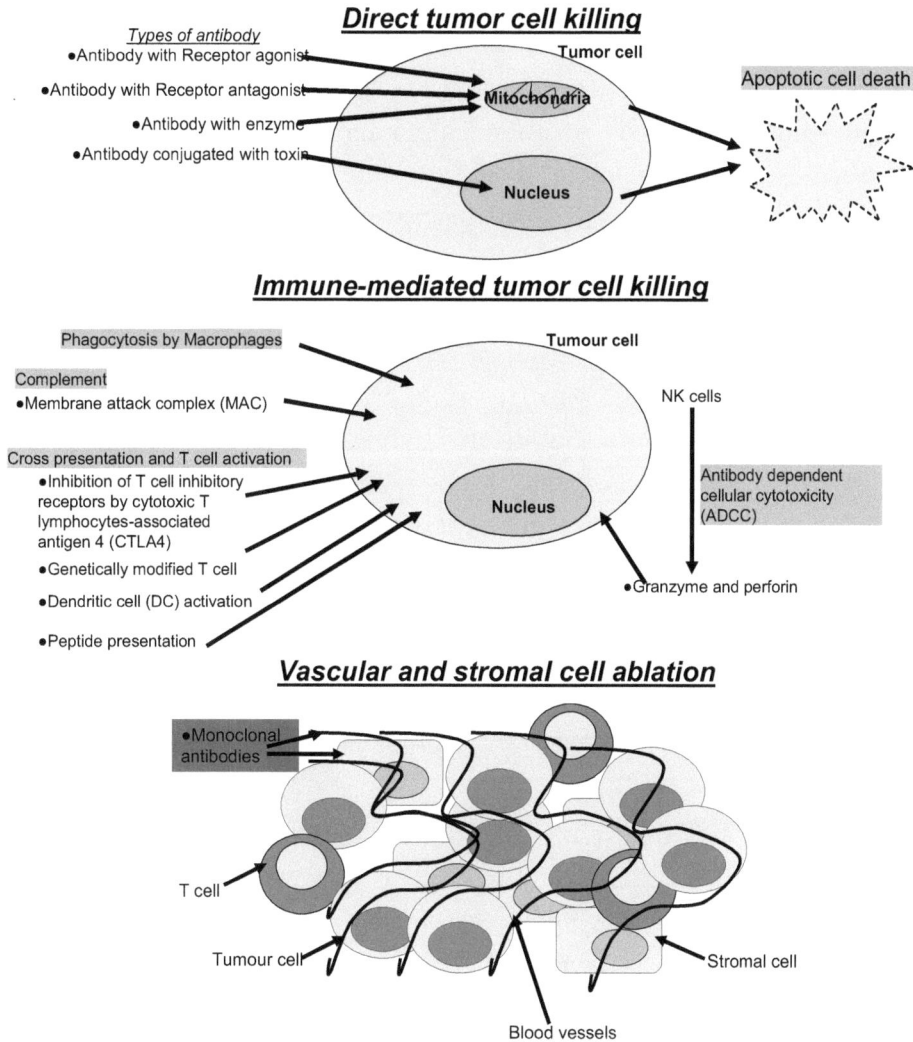

Fig. (1). Mechanism of tumor cell killing by antibodies (Modified from Scott *et al.*, 2012)

Immune mediated tumor cell killing includes induction of phagocytosis, complement activation, antibody-dependent cell-mediated cytotoxicity (ADCC), target gene-modified T cells and activation of T cells either through inhibition of T cell inhibitory receptors such as CTLA-4, or antibody-mediated cross presentation of antigen to dendritic cells (DCs). The Fc portion of antibodies is important for mediating tumor cell killing through CDC and ADCC [6, 16, 20]. Vascular and stromal ablation include vessel receptor antagonism or ligand trap, stromal cell inhibition and conjugated antibody delivery [19, 20].

The US Food and Drug Administration (FDA) has approved more than a dozen mAbs to treat solid tumors and hematological malignancies (Table **2**). In addition to these antibodies, a large number of mAbs are currently being tested in early and late-stage clinical trials. Some of these are discussed below:

Naked Monoclonal Antibodies

Naked monoclonal antibodies are the most commonly used mAbs to treat cancer. Characteristic feature of these mAbs is that no drug or radioactive materials are attached to them. Most mAbs attach to the antigens expressed on cancer cells. However, they also bind to antigens on non-cancerous cells and free floating proteins. Different mAbs function in different ways.

Alemtuzumab (Campath®)

One type of mAb boosts a person's immune system against cancer cells by attaching to them and acts as a marker for the body's immune system to destroy them. Example of such type of antibody is alemtuzumab (Campath®). It is a naked humanized IgG1 monoclonal antibody. It is used to treat patients with chronic lymphocytic leukemia (CLL), cutaneous T-cell lymphoma, peripheral T- cell lymphoma and T-cell prolymphocytic leukemia. Alemtuzumab binds to the CD52 antigen expressed on both T lymphocytes and B lymphocytes. CD52 is also expressed on monocytes. On binding to CD52, alemtuzumab initiates its cytotoxic effect by complement fixation and antibody dependent cell-mediated cytotoxicity (ADCC) mechanisms, thus involving the immune cells in destroying the cancer cells [1, 20].

Table 2. Therapeutic monoclonal antibodies approved by FDA [1, 20].

Immunotherapy (generic name)	Targets	Type of cancer treated
Unconjugated antibodies		
Rituximab	CD20	Non-Hodgkin lymphoma
Tastuzumab	HER2	Breast cancer
Alemtuzumab	CD52	Chronic lymphocytic leukaemia
Cetuximab	EGFR	Colorectal cancer

(Table 2) contd.....

Immunotherapy (generic name)	Targets	Type of cancer treated
Bevacizumab	VEGF-A	Colorectal, breast and lung cancer
Panitumumab	EGFR	Colorectal cancer
Ofatumumab	CD20	Chronic lymphocytic leukaemia
Immunoconjugates		
Gemtuzumab ozogamicin	CD33	Acute myelogenus leukemia
90Y-Ibritumomab tiuxetan	CD20	Lymphoma
Tositumomab and 131I-tositumomab	CD20	Lymphoma

Ipilimumab (Yervoy®)

It is a human IgG1 antibody that reacts with cytotoxic T-lymphocyte antigen-4 (CTLA-4). CTLA-4 plays critical role in the activation of T-reg cells that suppress the immune response. Under normal physiological condition, T cells are activated by two signals: (i) T cell receptors attached to the antigen-MHC complex and (ii) T-cell surface receptor CD28 attached to CD80 or CD86 on the surface of APCs. CTLA-4 binds to CD80 or CD86 and prevents binding of CD28 to these surface proteins, thereby inhibiting the activation of T cells [21].

Ipilimumab causes a shift in the ratio of regulatory T cells (Tregs) to cytotoxic T cells (CTLs). Since Treg cells inhibit the activation of other T cells, increasing the cytotoxic T cells and decreasing the Treg cells is one of the mechanisms by which this antibody functions. It is used to treat metastatic melanoma [21]

Bevacizumab (Avastin®)

Bevacizumab is a humanized IgG1 mAb that binds to and neutralizes the vascular endothelial growth factor (VEGF) ligand. It is used as a targeted therapy. VEGF is the central mediator of tumor angiogenesis and is produced by malignant cells. Bevacizumab functions by blocking the ligand that activates the VEGF receptor on tumor vessels. It also helps the chemotherapy to concentrate at the tumor site. Bevacizumab in combination with fluoropyrimidine-based chemotherapy is used in the first-line therapy of metastatic colorectal cancer and glioblastoma. It is also used to treat metastatic lung cancer, metastatic breast cancer and metastatic renal cancer [20, 21].

Cetuximab (Erbitux®)

Cetuximab is an anti-EGFR chimeric mAb which is used to treat patients with colorectal cancer. Its anti-tumor effects are primarily mediated by interfering with signal- transduction pathways that are activated by the surface antigen. EGFR is over-expressed in the vast majority of epithelial tumors. Its over expression is associated with increased proliferation, resistance to apoptosis and increased VEGF expression. Binding of cetuximab to EGFR blocks phosphorylation and activation of several tyrosine kinases that are associated with the receptor, thereby disrupting signal transduction that are associated with increased cell proliferation and resistance to apoptosis [21].

Ofatumumab (Arzerra®)

It is a second generation human IgG1 antibody that binds to CD20. Ofatumumab is used to treat chronic lymphocytic leukemia (CLL) where the B lymphoma cells express CD20 protein. The drug induces complement-dependent cytotoxicity [21].

Panitumumab (Vactibix®)

It is a fully human IgG2 antibody that became the first fully human mAb for cancer therapy. It binds to the extracellular domain of EGFR causing internalization of the receptor and antibody and disruption of downstream signal transductions that are associated with enhanced cell proliferation and resistance to apoptosis. The Ab is used as a single agent in refractory metastatic colorectal cancer [21].

Rituximab (Rituxan®)

It is a mouse-human chimeric monoclonal IgG1 antibody specific for CD20. Rituximab was the first mAb approved to treat human malignancy based on a high rate of durable response in patients with relapsed indolent B-cell lymphoma. Recombinant technology is used to produce this antibody. Rituximab is used to treat aggressive lymphomas such as diffuse large B-cell lymphoma and follicular lymphoma, and leukemia such as B cell chronic lymphocytic leukemia. Immunotherapy mechanisms by which this antibody attributes to tumor cell killing includes both complement mediated cytotoxicity (CMC) and antibody dependent cell-mediated cytotoxicity (ADCC), apoptosis and cellular senescent. Rituximab also increases sensitivity of cancerous cells to chemotherapy drugs and is the current standard induction treatment for follicular lymphoma [21].

Trastuzumab (Herceptin®)

Trastuzumab (Herceptin®) is another type of humanized naked mAb. mAb of this type works by attaching to and blocking antigens that signal the cancer cells to grow and spread. Example of this type of mAb is trastuzumab (Herceptin®). It is an antibody that reacts with human epidermal growth factor-2 (HER2). HER2 is expressed on the surface of some type of cancer such as breast and stomach cancer cells. Activation of HER2 helps the cancer cells to grow. Trastuzumab binds to these proteins and inhibits their activation [21].

Conjugated Monoclonal Antibodies

Conjugated monoclonal antibodies (mAbs) are coupled to a chemotherapy drug, toxin or radioactive particle, and hence are called conjugated monoclonal antibody. This type of mAb is used as homing device to carry the coupled substances to the cancer cells. The mAb circulates in the body until it finds an antigen on which it attaches. The attached mAb then delivers the toxic substance where it is needed most, thereby reducing the damage to the surrounding normal cells. Conjugated monoclonal Abs are also known as tagged, labelled, or loaded antibodies. They can be divided into several groups depending on what they are linked to [19].

Radiolabeled Antibodies

These mAbs have small radioactive particles attached to them. Treatment with radiolabeled antibody is also known as radioimmunotherapy (RIT). Example of some of these Abs are as follows:

Yttrium-90 Ibritumomab Tiuxetan (Zevalin®)

It is a mAb that functions by attaching to CD20 antigen, which is found on the cancerous B lymphocytes. The antibody delivers radioactive material directly to the cancerous B lymphocytes and is used to treat some types of non-Hodgkin lymphoma [19, 22].

Iodine-131 Tositumomab (Bexxar®)

This Ab is produced by direct iodination of tyrosine amino acids on the murine anti-CD20 mAb tositumomab. I-131 emits both γ radiation and β radiation with a half-life of 8 days. Only the β radiation has therapeutic importance. Tositumomab is used to treat indolent B-cell lymphoma [20, 23].

Chemolabeled Antibodies

These mAbs have chemotherapy or other drugs attached to them. These are also known as antibody-drug conjugates (ADCs). Some FDA approved chemolabeled antibodies are Brentuximab vedotin (Adcetris®) and Ado- trastuzumab emtansine (Kadcyla®, also called TDM-1) [20, 23].

Brentuximab vedotin is an antibody that targets the CD30 antigen found on lymphocytes, attached to a chemo drug called MMAE. This drug is used to treat Hodgkin lymphoma and anaplastic large cell lymphoma that do not respond to other treatments [20, 23]. Ado-trastuzumab emtansine is an antibody that is attached to a chemo drug called DM1. The Ab is used to treat advanced staged breast cancer patients and targets HER2 protein expressed on these cancerous cells [20, 23].

Toxin attached Antibodies

Denileukin diftitox (Ontak®) is a genetically engineered mAb which is a fusion product that consists of IL-2 attached to diphtheria endotoxin, thereby producing the immunotoxin DAB389IL-2. The diphtheria toxin-receptor binding domain is replaced with IL-2 to target IL-2 receptor. Although IL-2 is not an antibody, it attaches to certain cells in the body that contain the CD25 antigen, which makes it useful for delivering the immunotoxin into these cells. Once endocytosed into acidic vesicles, the toxin is released and inhibits protein synthesis resulting in cell death within few minutes. Denileukin diftitox is used to treat one type of skin cancer known as cutaneous T-cell lymphoma [20, 23].

Bispecific Monoclonal Antibodies

These antibodies are made up of parts of two different mAbs and can attach to two different proteins at the same time. Blinatumomab (Blincyto®) is used to treat acute lymphocytic leukemia (ALL). One part of blinatumomab attaches to the CD19 protein which is expressed on some leukemic and lymphoma cells. Another part of this antibody attaches to CD3 protein which is expressed on T cells. By attaching to both these proteins, blinatumomab brings both the cancer cells and immune cells together and is thought to induce the immune system to attack the cancer cells [20].

CANCER VACCINES

Cancer vaccines, also known as specific immunotherapy or cellular therapy are used either to treat an existing cancer or prevent cancer. Vaccines that are used to treat existing cancer are called therapeutic vaccines. Therapeutic cancer vaccines can be used to enhance endogenous immune response against the host's malignancy. Vaccine approaches use presentation of tumor antigens by antigen presenting cells (APCs) to enhance the tumor immune response or induce an antitumor immune response against a specific cancer. The technique involves removal of immune cells from blood or separation of antigens from tumor cells. Immune cells specific to the tumor antigen are activated, cultured and returned to the patients where the activated immune cells attack and kill cancer cells. The goal is to initiate an active immune response towards the tumor cell to kill the cancer cells. Immune cells that can be used include natural killer cells, lymphokine-activated killer cells, cytotoxic T cells and dendritic cells (DCs). Therapeutic cancer vaccines are available to treat breast, lung, colon, skin, kidney, prostate and other types of cancer. However, till now, only Provenge, a cell-based therapy has been approved to treat prostrate cancer [3, 21].

The other type of cancer vaccines that received regulatory approval are of preventive type. These are designed to prevent virus induced cancers. Studies showed that approximately 15% of all cancers are virally induced [3, 21].

Viral Vaccines

Human papilloma virus (HPV) causes cervical, anal, throat and other types of cancer. Two vaccines are available to treat HPV. These vaccines induce a humoral immune response against these serotypes of HPV. These vaccines target the human papilloma virus (HPV) serotypes HPV-16 and HPV-18. These vaccines are approved for administration in young girls. However, the vaccine is not effective if chronic HPV infection due to genomic integration of viral genes encoding oncoproteins E6 and E7 occurs [1, 23]. Overlapping synthetic long peptides from HPV-16 E6 and E7 oncoproteins in incomplete Freund's adjuvant have been used to vaccinate HPV-associated vulvar intraepithelial neoplasia Grade III (VINIII) [1, 23].

Another viral vaccine that showed promising results in Phase II trials is attenuated herpes simplex virus type. Herpes simplex virus (HSV) infects both healthy and tumor cells, but it multiplies in cancer cells only. After the virus destroys cancer cells, it releases tumor antigens that can be taken up by professional antigen-presenting cells. The virus can also induce systemic antitumor immune response from distinct sites or undergo another replication cycle in neighboring cancer cells.

The attenuated virus used for vaccine development is genetically modified to produce granulocyte-colony stimulating factor (GM-CSF). Trade name of the vaccine is OncoVex, BioVex. This oncolytic immunotherapeutic agent is injected into tumor cells. These vaccines are currently being used for the treatment of melanoma and head and neck squamous cell carcinoma [1, 23].

Vaccine-based immunotherapy against other virally induced cancer such as hepatitis B and Hepatitis C virus-induced hepatocellular carcinomas and Epstein-Barr virus (EBV)-associated nasopharyngeal carcinomas can be developed as the vaccine can be directed against viral proteins [1, 23].

Therapeutic Vaccines

Dendritic Cell Vaccines

Dendritic cells (DCs) are a discrete leukocyte population in the monocyte/macrophage family. DCs display antigen in the context of histocompatibility antigens to T-lymphocytes. DCs are known as professional antigen presenting cells (APCs) and they are able to take in, process and present antigen, are able to migrate through tissues and are able to stimulate antigen-specific T-cell responses. DCs are able to drive both CD4+ and CD8+ antigenic responses. Immature DCs are phagocytic and process antigens. However, as they mature, their phagocytic capacity and association with antigen presentation diminishes. Due to this property, DCs are of interest for antigen presentation for immunization or vaccination purposes for a primary response or to boost weak existing responses. Cytokines like IL-4 and the combination of IL-4 and GM-CSF optimize the production of DCs [24, 25].

DCs express a variety of cluster designation (CD) markers such as CD11c, CD80 (B7.1), CD86 (B7.2) and CD83 are used to define and characterize DCs and to differentiate between mature and immature DCs. CD80 and CD86 bind to CD28 for a co-stimulatory signal and to CTLA-4 for an inhibitory signal. Therefore, antigen loaded DCs are capable of producing either an anti-antigen immune response or tolerance. Dendritic cell receptors such as TLR3, TLR7, TLR8 or CD40 have also been used as targets by antibodies to produce immune responses [24, 25].

DCs have been administered by various routes. However, from product classification standpoint, these are considered as adoptive immunotherapy if pure DC populations without an antigen-loaded are administered. DCs with antigen-loaded and administered by s.c., i.d., intranodal, or lymphatic routes of administration are considered as vaccines. DCs are also used as adoptive immunotherapy. DCs are also used as adoptive immunotherapy [24, 25].

Sipuleucel-T (Provenge®) is a therapeutic vaccine and is designed to treat prostate cancer. It has been approved by the US Food and Drug Administration (FDA) to treat cancer. Although this vaccine does not cure cancer completely, it helps extend patient's life by several months on an average [26, 27]. Sipuleucel-T preparation involves several steps. At first immune cells are removed from the patient's blood and taken to a lab where the cells are treated with chemicals to turn intodendritic cells (DCs). These are then exposed to a protein called prostatic acid phosphatase (PAP), which produces an immune response against prostate cancer. These DCs are then introduced back into the patient by infusion into a vein (IV). The process is repeated twice more and two weeks apart so that the patient gets three doses of cells. Back in the body, the DCs influence other cells of the immune system to attack the prostate cancer cells [26, 27].

Adoptive Cellular Therapy

This involves the administration of cells as anticancer therapy. The approach involves *ex vivo* manipulation to enrich a particular cell type and/or to enhance cell activity. Different types of adoptive cellular therapies are available. These are: (i) natural killer cells and lymphokine-activated killer cells; (ii) tumor infiltrating lymphocytes and cytotoxic T-lymphocytes: (iii) CD3 driven helper T-lymphocytes; and (iv) non- myeloablative allogenic stem-cell transplant and donor lymphocyte infusions [26, 27].

Sipuleucel-T (Provenge®) is also considered as an adoptive cellular therapy. Another adoptive cellular therapy that received regulatory approval for cancer therapy is nonmyelablative allogenic bone-marrow transplant [26, 27].

Idiotype Vaccines for B-cell Malignancies

BiovaxID is a therapeutic cancer vaccine. It is an Orphan drug and received FDA approval with Phase III clinical trials. BiovaxID is used to treat follicular lymphoma (one type of non-Hodgkin's lymphoma). It is a personalized vaccine and manufactured from tissue biopsy obtained from a patient's tumor. This approach uses the expression of idiotype which is an epitope at the V region of B-cell lymphoma. Immunization with specific idiotypes produces endogenous human anti-idiotype antibodies and idiotype-specific cytotoxic CTL responses. Hybridoma and recombinant DNA techniques are used to rescue the idiotype from fresh lymphoma cells, followed by mass production for therapeutic use [1, 27].

IMMUNOTHERAPY IN DEVELOPMENT

Several immunotherapies are under development (Table **3**). Mentionable are discussed below:

Table 3. Immunomodulatory immunotherapies that are at the development stage/FDA approved as monotherapies [1].

Immunotherapy	Targets	Target expressing immune cells	Development stage
Daclizumamb	CD25	Tregs and activated T cells	Phase III
CT011, MDX-1106	PD-1	Activated T cells	Phase II
BMS-663513	CD137	NK cells, NKT cells, DCs, neutrophils and monocytes	Phase II
TRX518	GITR	Tregs cells	Phase I
Dacetuzumab	CD40	DCs, B cells, monocytes and macrophages	Phase I

Adoptive T-cell Therapy

This is a form of passive immunization involving transfusion of T-cells. These are found in blood and tissue and are activated in response to a foreign pathogen. These T cells are activated when the cells encounter other cells that display small part of foreign proteins on their surface antigens. These can be either infected cells or the antigen presenting cells (APCs). Those cells that are found in tumor tissues are known as tumor infiltrating lymphocytes (TILs). They are activated by the presence of APCs, mostly the dendritic cells (DCs) that present tumor antigens. However, within the tumor microenvironment, the cells of the immune system remain immunosuppressed, which prevents immune-mediated tumor death [26, 27].

Tumor targeted T cells are produced in several ways. T-cells (TILs) specific to a tumor antigen can be isolated from blood or tumor samples and then activated by suing gene therapy or by exposing the T cells to tumor antigens. Complete remission of leukemia was reported in two small clinical trials using this approach, although no adoptive T cell therapy has been approved yet [26, 27].

Another approach of adoptive transfer is haploidentical γδ T cells or NK cells from a healthy donor. Although these do not cause GvHD (graft-*versus*-host disease), the transferred cells show frequently impaired functions [26, 27].

Targeting Immunomodulatory Molecules

A number of naturally occurring molecule inhibit the antitumor immune response system and help the tumor cells in immune escape mechanism. These molecules can be used for therapeutic intervention [17]. Some of these molecules are discussed below:

Immune Checkpoint Blockade

Several monoclonal antibodies (mAbs) can be used as immunomodulatory antibodies, which are also known as immune checkpoint blockade (Table **3**). Immune checkpoint blockade refers to blockade of immune system inhibitory checkpoints. Immune checkpoints are either stimulatory or inhibitory. Blockade of inhibitory immune checkpoints activates the immune system function. For example, Abs targeting the suppressive co-stimulatory receptors CTLA-4 or PD-1 on T cells blocks inhibitory signals that are transmitted through these receptors and prolong the life of activated T cells [5].

Inhibitory Immune Checkpoints

<ins>*CTLA-4*</ins>

CTLA-4 is expressed on both CD4 and CD8 T cells, and the Treg or FOXP3+ regulatory T cells. Binding of CTLA4 to its ligands (B7-1 or CD80 and B7-2 or CD86) on antigen-presenting cells (APCs) inhibits activation of T cells. In this way CTLA-4 negatively regulates the activity of effector T cells. CTLA-4 out-competes the co-stimulation molecule CD28 for binding B7 molecules on APCs which results in delivery of inhibitory signals. Therefore, CTLA-4 controls T cell response. CTLA-4 is also constitutively expressed by Tregs for immune suppression of DCs when binding through B7. In humans, anti-CTLA-4 targets effector T cells only [5].

CTLA-4 specific mAbs target the T cell surface protein cytotoxic T lymphocyte-associated antigen 4 (CTLA-4). Two fully humanized antibodies have been developed that target CTLA-4. These are tremelimumab (by Pfizer) and ipilimumab (by Bristol-Myers Squibb). Ipilimumab, recently approved by the FDA, is used for second line treatment of metastatic melanoma. Tremelimumab is in development for the treatment of melanoma and other malignant diseases [5].

PD1

PD-1 (programmed death 1) is a member of the CD28 superfamily. The protein is upregulated on T cells upon activation. It is a suppressive regulator of T cell activity. The receptor PD1 is expressed on activated T cells, B cells, NK cells and Treg cells. PD1 has two identified ligands: PDL1 (also known as B7-H1) and PDL2 (also known as B7-DC). The receptors for PD-1, PD-1L and PD-2L, are normally expressed on self-cells to prevent autoimmunity. PDL1 has affinity for CD80. PDL1 is expressed on many solid tumors and is associated with poor prognosis. PD-1L is upregulated in a number of tumors, thereby inhibiting anti-tumor T cell responses. Accordingly, tumor infiltrating CD8+ T cells and CD4+ T cells show increased expression of PD-1 and are anergic.

Antibodies that inhibit the interaction between PD1 and its ligands are promising therapeutic interventions. PD1-specific agents include nivolumab, pembrolizumab and pidilizumab. PDL1-specific agents include atezolizumab, MEDI4736 and MSB0010718C; and PDL2-specific agents include rHIgM12B7 [5].

LAG3

Lymphocyte activation gene 3 protein (LAG3; also known as CD223) is progressively expressed on T cells during depletion. Until recently, the only ligand identified for LAG3is the major histocompatibility complex (MHC) class II molecules. The expression of LAG3 on tumor-infiltrating Treg cells and CTLs may be involved in immune evasion by tumors. BMS-986016, a LAG3-specific mAb, which is in clinical development to block LAG3, is thought to reverse T cell depletion and enhance antitumor immunity [5].

TIM3

T cell immunoglobulin and mucin domain-containing 3 (TIM3; also known as HAVCR2) is expressed on Th1 cells, CTLs and DCs. Its function differs depending on its expression on the cell type. TIM3 is expressed by tumor-infiltrating lymphocytes (TILs) in melanoma and non-small-cell lung cancer (NSCLC). TIM3 may be involved in lymphocyte inactivation or can induce apoptosis upon ligation to galectin 9. Its functional interaction with carcinoembryonic antigen-related cell adhesion molecule 1 (CEACAM1) has been studied too [5].

Co-stimulatory Receptors

CD137

CD137 CD137 is known as 4-1BB and TNFRSF9. It is a potent T cell and NK cell co-stimulatory receptor which is expressed at the cell surface of activated lymphocytes. Its signaling improves cytotoxic antitumor responses and T cell survival. Urelumab and PF-05082566 are agonistic CD137-specific mAbs that are under evaluation for different types of malignancies.

Agonistic CD137-specific mAbs may enhance NK cell-mediated antibody-dependent cellular cytotoxicity (ADCC). Data from mouse models studies showed that tumor cells coated with tumor- targeted mAbs induced the upregulation of CD137 expression on NK cells and subsequent addition of the agonist CD137-specific mAb increased NK cell degranulation causing tumor lysis. Preclinical synergistic effect was observed when CD137-specific mAbs was combined with rituximab (mAb specific for CD20), trastuzumab (mAb specific for human epidermal growth factor receptor 2 HER2; also known as ERBB2) or cetuximab (mAb specific for epidermal growth factor receptor (EGFR) [1, 17].

GITR

GITR (glucocorticoid induced tumor necrosis factor TNF receptor, TNFRSF18) is a constitutively expressed co-stimulatory molecule on Treg cells and effector T cells. Co-stimulation of CD3 and GITR results in proliferation of both Tregs and effector T cells. The expanded Tregs are functionally unresponsive, while the effector T cells gain functional activity. GITR reverses Treg cell-mediated suppression of T cells and activates proliferation and effector functions in CD4+ and CD8+ T cells. Activated GITR may overcome self-tolerance, reverse Treg cell-mediated suppression and enhance antitumor immune responses. The agonistic GITR-specific mAbs TRX518 and MK-4166 are undergoing Phase I evaluation [1, 15].

OX40

OX40, also known as TNFRSF4 is a co-stimulatory receptor expressed primarily on activated CD4+ and CD8+ T cells. It enhances anti-tumor immune responses by promoting T cell proliferation and survival. Preclinical studies using mouse model studies showed that OX40 agonists enhanced antitumor immunity by inhibiting Treg cells and promoting T cell survival. Several agonistic OX40-specific mAbs are under clinical evaluation [1, 15].

CD40

CD40, also known as TNFRSF5, is a stimulatory surface receptor of the tumor necrosis factor receptor (TNFR) family. CD40 promotes the activation of APCs and enhances their co-stimulatory and antigen presentation activities, leading to T cell activation. CD40 enables APCs to prime CD8+ T cell differentiation. An agonistic CD40-specific antibody is under evaluation [1, 17].

CD27

CD27 is a receptor of the TNFR superfamily which is expressed on resting and naive T lymphocytes but not on fully differentiated effector T cells. The receptor is also expressed on a subset of NK cells. Binding of CD27 to its ligand, CD70, on activated APCs enhances T cell activation, effector function, maturation, survival and long-term memory of the CD27-expressing cell. CD27 has a role in enhancing NK cell proliferation and cytotoxicity, in B cell activation and immunoglobulin synthesis. CDX-1127, a CD27-directed mAb, is under clinical development. [1, 15].

Killer Inhibitory Receptors

Inhibitory killer cell immunoglobulin (Ig)-like receptors (KIRs) negatively regulate the cytotoxic activities of NK cells and some T cell subsets. KIRs recognize self-MHC class I molecules on cells and can inhibit NK cell activation. The loss or downregulation of self-MHC class I molecules observed in most tumor cells is sufficient to induce NK cell sensitivity. However, many tumor cells retain proper MHC class I expression that can evade immune surveillance by NK cells and escape immune-mediated destruction. The use of KIR- specific mAbs for cancer therapy is under evaluation. Lirilumab is a pan-specific KIR mAb designed to block multiple KIR family members. NK cells and certain T lymphocyte subsets express other cytotoxicity-inhibiting receptors, such as NKG2A and CD96, which are also potential targets for cancer immunotherapy [1, 15].

Combination Therapy

Immunotherapy drugs as monotherapy may be less effective in tumor regression. Therefore, multiple strategies for eliciting and enhancing antitumor immunity have been developed and some are in clinical use. At present, much focus has been given to synergistic immunotherapy combining different immunotherapies or combining immunotherapies with other treatment modalities of cancer. Two parameters define synergy in cancer immunotherapy: (i) the intensity of the elicited measureable immune response against cancer; and (ii) the actual reduction or disappearance of tumor lesions. Preclinical and clinical synergies have also been observed for immuno-oncology agents in combination with chemotherapy, targeted therapies, radiotherapy, anti-angiogenic agents and partial surgical resections. Two most studied fields are use of immunomodulatory or signaling molecules and the other one is adoptive T cell therapy [17]. Here, we discuss a number of synergistic combinations that stem from pre-clinical studies and lead to stepwise testing in humans.

Combining Immune Checkpoint Inhibitors

Combination therapies that are used to block more than one immunomodulatory pathway can enhance the anti-tumor efficacy of each individual treatment.

Combination of CTLA-4 specific and PD1-specific inhibitory mAbs showed marked antitumor activity in some tumor models. These negative regulators affect different signaling pathways within T cells, and therefore can be used synergistically for therapeutic purpose, more specifically through enhancing CTL effector activity [15].

Combination of anti-PD-1 treatment and a GM-CSF secreting whole cell vaccine significantly prolonged mice challenged with B16 melanoma or with CT26 colon cancer. The combined blockade of both PD-1 and CTLA-4 was found to synergize with a vaccine that was used to treat B16-B6 melanoma tumors. The synergistic effect on tumor growth lead to increased tumor infiltration of CD8+ T cells expressing CTLA-4 and PD-1. Dual blockade of PD-1 and CTLA-4 signaling eliminates T cell suppressive mechanisms [17]. This combination increases longevity of T cells. An alternate mechanism for the synergistic effect of combined PD-1 and CTLA-4 blockade is by inhibition of MDSC suppression. This was tested in mice bearing I8D ovarian tumors where elevated levels of both PD-1 and CTLA-4 were observed. Administration of the blocking antibodies *in vitro* resulted reduced levels of arginase I activity in MDSCs. Arginase I is a mechanism through which MDSCs attenuate T cell activation [15].

Combination of ipilimumab and nivolumab stimulates the combinations of other immune checkpoint inhibitors preclinically and clinically. Combinations of PD1-specific antibodies with specific antibodies against LAG3 or TIM3 showed synergistic PD1 blockade in mouse tumor models [15]. Another interesting combination approach involved delivering immuno-stimulatory mAbs with immune checkpoint inhibitors. A Phase I–II trial is underway to evaluate a combination of PD1-blocking agents with CD137-specific mAbs. However, these may pose new challenges for the clinical management of patient's safety [15].

The combination of tremelimumab and the CD40-specific superagonist antibody CP-870,893 is also being examined in patients with metastatic melanoma [15].

In addition, trials are ongoing in patients with advanced-stage solid tumors to evaluate the combination of OX40-specific mAbs with checkpoint inhibitors (MEDI6469) plus tremelimumab or MEDI4737, and that of lirilumab with nivolumab or ipilimumab [15].

Current knowledge of the crosstalk among co-inhibitory and co-stimulatory receptors is limited. Multiple mechanisms for synergy arise when considering that the functions repressed by checkpoints are frequently induced by co-stimulatory molecules on the same target cells. At present, combinations of mAbs targeting co-stimulatory molecules (such as CD137-specific and GITR-specific antibodies) with PD1-specific or PDL1-specific antibodies work synergistically in mouse models, but it is difficult to predict the effect in human. Therefore, these combinations should be evaluated carefully in early clinical trials [15].

Combining Immunomodulation with Chemotherapies

Conventional treatment regimens include chemotherapy, radiotherapy and targeted therapy. These therapies induce ADCC mediated immune response. Here, we discussed some of the synergistic effects that were observed combining immunomodulatory mAbs with the combination of the conventional immunotherapy, particularly chemotherapy (Table **4**) [14].

Chemotherapies have the potential to enhance cancer vaccine-induced immune suppression through several mechanisms. These include: (i) targeting the immune system to reduce tumor–induced immune suppressive cells; (ii) targeting the tumor to increase immunogenicity by increasing MHC or antigen expression; and (iii) directly stimulating effector response by activating T cells [14]. Some recent studies showed that combination of chemotherapy after vaccination may be a better treatment schedule than chemotherapy pre-treatment or concurrent treatment (Table 3). In a clinical study, patients with extensive stage small cell lung cancer (NSCLC) were found to be more responsive to second-line chemotherapy treatment after vaccination with DCs transduced with wild-type p53 *via* adenoviral vector. In another study, NSCLC patients were treated with TG4010 viral vector encoding MUC1 and IL-2. However, the combination treatment was not optimal for all types of cancer treatment. For example, ovarian cancer patients who had previously received a p53-synthetic long peptide (SLP)® vaccine followed by chemotherapy treatment were not benefited from the combination treatment, although this startegy was beneficial to NSCLC patients [5].

Several strategies have been used to overpower tumor immune evasion and suppression mechanisms to accomplish a targeted approach like cancer vaccines combined with one or more chemotherapies to help lower tumor defences and boost the immune system. This could be achieved on three levels: (i) by increasing tumor visibility to the immune system through increased expression of MHC class I and unique surface antigens; (ii) decreasing tumor induced immune suppression; and (iii) increase T cell stimulation. Chemotherapies could condition both the immune system and the tumor so that the cancer vaccines have the best chance of success [5].

A number of chemotherapy drugs can induce the immune system. For example, cyclophsophamide (CPA) and paclitaxel (PA) can increase effector T cell stimulation *via* shifting the immune response towards Th1 after vaccination with GM-CSF-secreting whole cell vaccine. Doxorubicin (DR) can increase tumor immunogenicity by inducing the immunologic death of tumor cells. 5-fluoruracil (5FU) and cisplatin can increase tumor immunogenicity by causing an upregulation of tumor-specific markers *in vitro* leading to increased recognition and killing by antigen-specific CD8 T cell lines. Cyclophsophamide (CPA) and gemcitabine (GEM) decrease tumor induced immune suppression caused by Tregs and MDSCs, respectively (ref: immunomodulation of chemotherapy). Paclitaxel (PX) induces tumor apoptosis by arresting cells undergoing mitosis. PX treatment could be used as a complementary drug to a survivin-targeted vaccine. Survivin is an anti-apoptotic protein that is upregulated by many types of cancers. Surviving-based peptide vaccines have been studied in several pre-clinical and clinical trials. PX treatment not only induces immunologic death of tumors but could also increase the expression of the vaccine target [5].

Combination of ipilimumab either with a GP100 peptide vaccine or with the chemotherapeutic agent dacarbazine showed that the first combination did not add toxicity or benefit to ipilimumab alone, but the dacarbazine and ipilimumab combination conferred a survival benefit to dacarbazine alone. Dacarbazine is a DNA-alkylating agent and causes tumor cell destruction through the release of antigens and senses immune cells of tumor-derived DNA. However, this combination was discontinued due to increased level of liver enzyme and hepatotoxicity. A different drug combination of ipilimumab with temozolomide (a drug similar in structure to dacarbazine) did not have such a high rate of dose-limiting liver toxicity, as unlike dacarbazine, temozolomide is not metabolized by the liver [5].

Hepatotoxicity was also reported when the BRAF-V600E inhibitor vemurafenib was combined with ipilimumab. Preclinical data in mice did not show any detrimental effect on their viability. However, clinical studies in human patients showed skin toxicity and liver toxicity, especially grade III elevation of liver enzymes in six of ten patients that were selected for the study [5].

Ipilimumab has also been combined with the vascular endothelial growth factor (VEGF) inhibitor bevacizumab. VEGF takes part in angiogenesis but it also has immune-modulating properties which include decreasing the influx of lymphocytes and DCs into the tumor, while increasing the intratumoral frequencies of Treg cells and myeloid-derived suppressor cells (MDSCs). A trial combining ipilimumab and bevacizumab in patients with metastatic melanoma showed that this combination and the efficacy was remarkably good, resulting in a median overall survival of more than 2 years. The combination showed an accumulation of CD8+ T cells and DCs in the tumor microenvironment [5].

Table 4. Immunotherapies that are in combination regimens and are in clinical trials [17].

Type of combination	Agents	Type of cancer	Overall response as combination regimen (CR and PR)
Immunotherapies	Ipilimumab and nivolumab	Advanced stage untreated melanoma	58%
		Advanced stage melanoma	42%
	Ipilimumab and bevacizumab	Advanced stage melanoma	19.6%
Immunotherapy and peptide vaccine	Ipilimumab and GP100 vaccine	Previously treated advanced stage melanoma	5.7%
Immunotherapy and chemotherapy	Ipilimumab and dacarbazine	Treatment-naïve advanced stage melanoma	15.2%
	Carboplatin plus paclitaxel and ipilimumab	NSCLC	32% irBORR ipilimumab
		ED-SCLC	71% irBORR ipilimumab

Combining granulocyte–macrophage colony-stimulating factor (GM-CSF) with ipilimumab showed synergistic antitumor activity through increased inflammation of the tumor. In a Phase II clinical trial that assessed the combination of ipilimumab and subcutaneous GM-CSF, the incidence and severity of immune-mediated adverse events associated with ipilimumab were unexpectedly mitigated by this combination. Results from this randomized study showed improved 1-year survival and overall survival in patients with metastatic melanoma In addition, gastrointestinal toxic effects were significantly less frequent and less severe in the combined treatment group compared with ipilimumab alone.

'CR' refers to complete response, 'PR' refers to partial response, and 'irBORR' refers to immune –related best overall response.

CONCLUSION

Immunotherapy drugs as monotherapy are less effective in inducing anti-tumor immune response. On the other hand, chemotherapy drugs have many side effects that are irreversible. Synergistic combination of immunotherapy and chemo-therapy can reduce dose associated toxicity.

Studies of combined PD1 and CTLA4 blockade in melanoma and other tumor types suggest that immune checkpoint inhibitors can be safely given to patients either as monotherapy or as combination therapy. Immunotherapy combinations can also reduce adverse events caused by monotherapy, despite that only a few combination/synergistic therapy are in clinical trial. A number of challenges exist with the therapy. One such challenge is managing combination-associated toxicity in synergistic application of the drugs. Most of the clinical studies of synergistic combination are translated from pre-clinical studies in mouse models. As a result, the consequences of the adverse effects of the combination of drugs are often unknown. In addition, checkpoint-targeted immunotherapies can induce a new class of adverse effects as a result of supraphysiological immune activation that may overwhelm key organ tolerance mechanisms. These immune-mediated adverse events mimic autoimmune diseases such as dermatitis, inflammatory colitis, thyroiditis, *etc.* Clinically apparent dermal and mucosal inflammation might also result from overactive immune responses to antigens of the common flora of the gut and induce gastrointestinal diseases. Each immunotherapeutic class of drugs is associated with adverse events that can be clinically managed, which is not feasible with the chemotherapy drugs all the time [17].

Another challenge in immunotherapy is the selection of the optimal patient population, and the optimal biological dose and schedule for immunotherapies are two major issues that still need to be resolved. With regard to the optimal patient population, patients with a minimal tumor burden are considered to have a better chance for response compared to patients with extensive and widespread disease. However, finding the optimal biological dose and schedule is much more complicated for immunotherapies than for classic chemotherapy. For most immunotherapies there is a lack of tools to select the best dose and schedule, and the decision to take a regimen to the ultimate test [3].

The challenges associated with immunotherapy as monotherapy or combination therapy require further studies on biomarker identification and reduction of toxicity is crucial to design effective combination immunotherapy. This can be achieved by implementing different technological platforms and integrating data to interpret the genotype and phenotypic relation so that these can be implemented in personalized medicines. In addition, the final interpretation of the data also requires technical experts from multidisciplinary background. In the next chapter, we will discuss these technological sites and their application in the field of cancer immunotherapy.

CONFLICT OF INTEREST

The author confirms that author has no conflict of interest to declare for this publication.

ACKNOWLEDGEMENTS

Decleared none.

REFERENCES

[1]   Lesterhuis WJ, Haanen JB, Punt CJ. Cancer immunotherapy--revisited. Nat Rev Drug Discov 2011; 10(8): 591-600.
[http://dx.doi.org/10.1038/nrd3500] [PMID: 21804596]

[2]   Margolin K, Lazarus M, Kaufman HL. Cytokines in the treatment of cancer. In: Curiel TJ, Ed. Cancer Immunother. Berlin, Germany: Springer 2013; pp. 173-210.
[http://dx.doi.org/10.1007/978-1-4614-4732-0_7]

[3]   Gajewski TF. Cancer immunotherapy. Mol Oncol 2012; 6(2): 242-50.

[http://dx.doi.org/10.1016/j.molonc.2012.01.002] [PMID: 22248437]

[4]   Ramkrishnan R, Gabrilovich DI. Mechanism of synergistic effect of chemotherap.pdf. Cancer Immunol Immunother 2011; 60: 419-23.
[http://dx.doi.org/10.1007/s00262-010-0930-1] [PMID: 20976448]

[5]   Weir GM, Liwski RS, Mansour M. Immune modulation by chemotherapy or immunotherapy to enhance cancer vaccines. Cancers (Basel) 2011; 3(3): 3114-42.
[http://dx.doi.org/10.3390/cancers3033114] [PMID: 24212948]

[6]   Scott AM, Wolchok JD, Old LJ. Antibody therapy of cancer. Nat Rev Cancer 2012; 12(4): 278-87.
[http://dx.doi.org/10.1038/nrc3236] [PMID: 22437872]

[7]   Lake RA, Robinson BW. Immunotherapy and chemotherapy--a practical partnership. Nat Rev Cancer 2005; 5(5): 397-405.
[http://dx.doi.org/10.1038/nrc1613] [PMID: 15864281]

[8]   Zitvogel L, Galluzzi L, Smyth MJ, Kroemer G. Mechanism of action of conventional and targeted anticancer therapies: reinstating immunosurveillance. Immunity 2013; 39(1): 74-88.
[http://dx.doi.org/10.1016/j.immuni.2013.06.014] [PMID: 23890065]

[9]   Nowak AK, Lake RA, Robinson BW. Combined chemoimmunotherapy of solid tumours: improving vaccines? Adv Drug Deliv Rev 2006; 58(8): 975-90.
[http://dx.doi.org/10.1016/j.addr.2006.04.002] [PMID: 17005292]

[10]   Lind MJ. Principles of cytotoxic chemotherapy. Syst Ther 2007; 36: 19-23.

[11]   BC Cancer Agency. Cancer Drug Manual [23 Dec 2013]. Available from: http://www.bccancer.bc.ca/HPI/DrugDatabase/default.htm

[12]   Rahman M, Chan AP, Tang M, Tai IT. A peptide of SPARC interferes with the interaction between caspase8 and Bcl2 to resensitize chemoresistant tumors and enhance their regression *in vivo*. PLoS One 2011; 6(11): e26390.
[http://dx.doi.org/10.1371/journal.pone.0026390] [PMID: 22069448]

[13]   Nowak AK, Lake RA, Robinson BW. Combined chemoimmunotherapy of solid tumours: improving vaccines? Adv Drug Deliv Rev 2006; 58(8): 975-90.
[http://dx.doi.org/10.1016/j.addr.2006.04.002] [PMID: 17005292]

[14]   Ramakrishnan R, Antonia S, Gabrilovich DI. Combined modality immunotherapy and chemotherapy: a new perspective. Cancer Immunol Immunother 2008; 57(10): 1523-9.
[http://dx.doi.org/10.1007/s00262-008-0531-4] [PMID: 18488219]

[15]   Hanahan D, Weinberg RA. Dendreon. Cancer Immunotherapy: fundamental concepts and emerging role. Oncol Perspect 2013; 100(1): 57-70.

[16]   Scott AM, Allison JP, Wolchok JD, Hughes H. Monoclonal antibodies in cancer therapy. Cancer Immun 2012; 12: 14.
[PMID: 22896759]

[17]   Melero I, Berman DM, Aznar MA, Korman AJ, Pérez Gracia JL, Haanen J. Evolving synergistic combinations of targeted immunotherapies to combat cancer. Nat Rev Cancer 2015; 15(8): 457-72.
[http://dx.doi.org/10.1038/nrc3973] [PMID: 26205340]

[18]   Shuptrine CW, Surana R, Weiner LM. Monoclonal antibodies for the treatment of cancer. Semin Cancer Biol 2012; 22(1): 3-13.
[http://dx.doi.org/10.1016/j.semcancer.2011.12.009] [PMID: 22245472]

[19]   Weiner LM, Dhodapkar MV, Ferrone S. Monoclonal antibodies for cancer immunotherapy. Lancet 2009; 373(9668): 1033-40.
[http://dx.doi.org/10.1016/S0140-6736(09)60251-8] [PMID: 19304016]

[20]   Hirschhorn-cymerman D, Perales M. Immunotherapy of Cancer 2010; 651: 131-55.
[http://dx.doi.org/10.1007/978-1-60761-786-0_9]

[21]   Weiner LM, Surana R, Wang S. Monoclonal antibodies: versatile platforms for cancer immunotherapy. Nat Rev Immunol 2010; 10(5): 317-27.
[http://dx.doi.org/10.1038/nri2744] [PMID: 20414205]

[22]   Finn OJ. Vaccines for cancer prevention: a practical and feasible approach to the cancer epidemic. Cancer Immunol Res 2014; 2(8): 708-13.
[http://dx.doi.org/10.1158/2326-6066.CIR-14-0110] [PMID: 25092812]

[23]   Palucka K, Banchereau J. Dendritic-cell-based therapeutic cancer vaccines. Immunity 2013; 39(1): 38-48.
[http://dx.doi.org/10.1016/j.immuni.2013.07.004] [PMID: 23890062]

[24]   Radford KJ, Tullett KM, Lahoud MH. Dendritic cells and cancer immunotherapy. Curr Opin Immunol 2014; 27: 26-32.
[http://dx.doi.org/10.1016/j.coi.2014.01.005] [PMID: 24513968]

[25]   Kalos M, June CH. Adoptive T cell transfer for cancer immunotherapy in the era of synthetic biology. Immunity 2013; 39(1): 49-60.
[http://dx.doi.org/10.1016/j.immuni.2013.07.002] [PMID: 23890063]

[26]   Ruella M, Kalos M. Adoptive immunotherapy for cancer. Immunol Rev 2014; 257(1): 14-38.
[http://dx.doi.org/10.1111/imr.12136] [PMID: 24329787]

[27]   Pejawar-Gaddy S, Finn OJ. Cancer vaccines: accomplishments and challenges. Crit Rev Oncol Hematol 2008; 67(2): 93-102.
[http://dx.doi.org/10.1016/j.critrevonc.2008.02.010] [PMID: 18400507]

CHAPTER 5

Systems Biology Approach in Cancer Immuno-therapy

Abstract: Systems biology is relatively a new field of study in cancer research. However, this approach has gained much attention as it can be used to understand the molecular level of a system under diseased or healthy condition and under dynamic or static condition. The approach allows understanding the interaction of DNA, RNA, protein and metabolite levels of a cell. Since, the cancer micro-environment consists of highly heterogeneous population of cells, systems biology is the robust tool that can be applied to understand this complex environment in the presence of perturbed condition using small molecules or targeted drugs like immunotherapy. Systems biology is already applied by drug design and discovery companies as well as by drug regulatory agencies to monitor safety and toxicity of the drug. The high throughput (HT) technological platforms generate un-biased datasets. However, data–mining is a problem for this approach. Despite this drawback, systems biology has been used in cancer immunotherapy to some extent. In this chapter, we discuss the known application of systems biology in cancer immunotherapy in particular to its application in biomarker identification, vaccine development, application in combination therapy, use in the development of validation models and future application in personalized medicine.

Keywords: Biomarkers, Drug discovery, Omics platforms, Personalized medicine, Systems biology.

INTRODUCTION

The field of immunotherapy is challenged by several factors. These include biomarker identification that correlates to the diseased state, target selection, animal model validation, decision on whether the drug should advance into phase III trial or not and placement of the drug in market by drug discovery and

Mahbuba Rahman

development company [1]. Overcoming these challenges requires the use of approaches which provides integrated information about different layers of a cell ranging from DNA to RNA to protein to metabolites. This eventually requires the involvement of broad group of professionals ranging from molecular biologists, immunologists, clinicians, bionformaticians, drug design and discovery companies and regulatory bodies. Systems biology is such an approach and over the last 25 years, it has been extensively used in different fields of life sciences research including drug design and discovery, biomarker identification of complex diseases such as cancer and autoimmune diseases, target validation and many other applications. The approach is also being considered for personalized medicine so that the treatment can be tailored to specific diseased group. The field of cancer immunotherapy belongs to drug design and discovery field [2]. As a result, many challenges faced by drug design and discovery company are common challenges for cancer immunotherapy field. In this chapter, we will discuss the challenges associated with immunotherapy development. Other challenges such as marketing, clinical trial and safety related issues will be discussed in chapter 6.

CHALLENGES IN CANCER IMMUNOTHERAPY

Challenges in Biomarker Identification

Detection of biomarkers in tumor environment may involve invasive repeated biopsies. Peripheral blood (PB) may be attractive to analyse some biomarkers. However, it may not reflect the local tumor microenvironment. In addition, potential biases may be introduced by the site of tumor collection. Samples of superficial cutaneous and lymph node metastases may be the easiest to collect, but their biology differs from the primary tumor and the metastatic sample. This also affects tumor staging. For example, PDL1 expression varies by melanoma location. Again, the location of metastases itself works as a prognostic marker. Visceral metastases are associated with a worse prognosis than non-visceral metastases [3, 4].

Another challenge is the assessment of tumor samples by flow cytometry (FC). FC is used to analyse functional information on specific immune cell types using cell suspensions. This is very difficult to carry out due to limited sample volume.

Accurate quantification can be carried out by using immunohistochemistry (IHC) and gene expression profiling technologies. However, incorporation of multi-colour tissue immunofluorescence can maximize the information obtained from limited biopsy specimens [3, 4].

Another technological challenge in biomarker identification is the application of serological analysis of recombinant cDNA expression libraries (SEREX) to identify cancer testis antigens, such as NY-ESO-1, and the MAGE, LAGE, GAGE families. SEREX involves the construction of cDNA expression libraries and protein expression followed by autologous serological screening for detecting reactivity of the proteins with antibodies present in the sera of the patient or subjects. Although this is a productive approach, it is a laborious technique and may not yield quantitative data [5].

Challenges with Combination Therapy

Two main types of combination regimens are under investigation. These include a combination of immunotherapies with standards of care and combination immunotherapies among themselves. However, combination therapy is challenged by several factors. Decision on the optimal immunotherapy combinations accurately requires the identification and validation of reliable surrogate biomarkers. In addition, confirmation on their clinical activity is also dependent on biomarker identification. Besides, new combinations into the clinic are to be informed by preclinical data in animal models and mechanistic evidence for pharmacodynamic interactions and selection of patients based on biomarkers primarily found in malignant tissue biopsies. However, only limited data are available on the information as which combination is the best for a given specific malignant indication or for a given patient and predictive models exist for clinicians. Therefore, scientists and clinicians need to work together actively in order to discover and develop new agents as partners for combination and take advantage of biotechnological advances, especially the systems biology approaches to produce improved, next-generation immuno-oncology agents. Consideration needs to be given to delivery routes of immunotherapies to maximize their bioavailability in tumors and tumor-draining lymph nodes, efficacy, specificity and toxicity that might be caused from the combination of the drugs. Agents with low efficacy as immunotherapy, but with multiplicative potential for synergistic effects, should also be tested. In addition, it will be important to consider the optimal types of trial design for combination therapies [3, 4].

Challenges with Animal Models

Animal models are used in pre-clinical studies to trace the effect of chemotherapy drug either as monotherapy or combination therapy. However, limitation of these models is that the observations do not always reflect the complex interactions between the human immune system and a heterogeneous tumor that has undergone immune-editing [3].

Systems biology approaches can help to mitigate some of the challenges that are currently observed in cancer immunotherapy fields. In the following sections, we discuss the technological platforms and the approaches of systems biology in the context of cancer immunotherapy studies followed by its applications in known areas of cancer immunotherapy [1, 6].

TECHNOLOGIES OF SYSTEMS BIOLOGY USED IN CANCER IMMUNOTHERAPY

Systems biology is a holistic approach, which integrates different levels of information in a cell quantitatively followed by mathematical and computational model development. Unlike reductionist approach which involves 'one gene' analysis, systems biology is an un-biased approach as it uses different high-throughput techniques. The ultimate goal is to understand the complex physiology of a cell under diseased or perturbed condition. The approach requires the capture and integration of measurements from multiple hierarchical levels of information ranging from DNA, RNA, protein-protein interactions, protein-DNA interactions and metabolites [8, 9].

System biology research encompasses wet experiment and dry experiment. The wet experiments include preparation and processing of biological samples and acquisition of raw datasets using high-throughput (HT) omics platforms (Table **1**). Different software tools are available that are relevant to the experiment and HT platforms. Once the raw data are acquired, these are further analyzed using different analysis tools which are mostly mathematical and computational tools. Analysis is the part of the dry experiment. Although HT platforms were used by immunologists for many years, downstream analysis of samples focusing resources from immunology and workflows has recently been incorporated (Table **2** and Table **3**) [10].

Table 1. Summary of high-throughput (HT) omics platforms used in systems biology and cancer immunotherapy [7].

Omics type	Description	Tools
Genomics	Comprehensive study on the genome of the organism. Information obtained from genome sequence helps to understand the function of genes.	Next generation sequencing (NGS) platforms (Illumina, SOLID, 454), deep sequencing, capillary sequencing, Sanger sequencing.
Transcriptomics	It is the expression level of mRNA under particular condition. The methods provide information on the protein-encoding messenger RNA transcripts and alternative spliced variants.	Affymetrix arrays, tiling arrays, PCR, RNA-Seq
Epigenetics	These are non-genomic encoded DNA modifications, including methylated CpG genomic sequences.	MethylCap-Seq and next-generation sequencing
miRNA	small, non-coding RNA molecules that regulate gene transcription via gene silencing	Microarray and RNA-Seq
Proteomics	The entire set of proteins, enzymes, receptors and structural units of the cell in a certain condition.	2D-PAGE gels, protein arrays, GC-MS, LC-MS, immuno-based methods; tissue microarray (TMA)
Phosphoproteomics	Protein phosphorylation at the post-translational modification level plays a key role in cell signaling	MS and immuno-based methods
Metabolomics	All the extracellular and intracellular metabolites including lipids, nucleotides, dipeptides and hormones produced under normal or diseased condition	Different quenching and extraction method, GC-MS, LC-MS, HPLC, spectrometric assay.
Fluxomics	Measures the combination of active metabolic fluxes in the cell under certain conditions. Flux analyses provide information about the activity of the pathways associated with perturbed condition.	13C labelling and analysis of enrichment patterns of proteinogenic amino acids using GC-MS / NMR.

Table 2. Resources for systems biology [7].

Resource type	Data source
Genomics	NCBI, GWAS
Transcriptomics	ArrayExpress, GEO, miRBase
Proteomics	Human Protein Reference Database (HPRD), Proteomics Identifications (PRIDE), UniProt
Phosphoproteomics	PhosphoSitePlus, Phosph.ELM, PTMcode
Metabolomics	Human Metabolome Database
Protein interaction databases	BioGRID, Database of Interacting Proteins, STRING, CORUM, PCDq
Pathway databases	KEGG, NCI Pathway Interaction Database, REACTOME
Tools for analysis and visualization	BioAssay Research Database, Bioconductor, BioGPS, BioPortal, cmap, Cytoscape FUnCoup, Ingenuity, Pathway Studio, OpenBEL, Database for Annotation, Visualization and Integrated Discovery

Table 3. Data analysis tools for immunology and immunotherapy [10].

Data type/tools	Program name
TCR repertoire	MiTCR, Decombinator, iSSAKE, IMGT, HIGHV-Quest
Antibody repertoire	IMGT, HIGHV-Quest, IgTree, VDJFasta
RNA-seq	VarScan, GATK, SAMtoos, ERANGE, Scripture, Cufflinks, CuffDiff, EdgeR, DESeq, Myrna, PoissonSeq
ChIP-seq	ERANGE, CisGenome, MACS, PeakSeq, SPP
eQTL	MatrixEQTL, PLINK, R/qtl, snpMatrix
Networks	WGCNA, coXpress, Inferelator, ARACNE, RimbaNET
Cytometry	FlowMeans, FLAME, FLOCK, SamSPECTRAL, SPADE, viSNE
Visualization	Cytoscape, Gephi, Circos
Online tools (databases)	ImMunoGenetics, Immport, MsigDB, GenePattern, DAVID, Stanford Data Miner, Structure, PCAdmix, myPEG, GWASdb, HaploReg, RegulomeDB, GRAIL, GSEA, ProfileChaser, LINCS browser

Analysis tools also use computational and mathematical modelings followed by the integration of the vast quantities of individual data points into molecular networks that underlie the biology of the system. These eventually develop hypothetical models, which are then tested and validated in experimental animals or tissue culture to tie the phenotype with the protein and gene regulatory networks [8, 11]. Here we discuss some of the systems biology tools that are used in cancer immunology and immunotherapy fields.

Genomics

Genomic technologies are used to define sequence, sequence variation and gene expression and manipulate genetic sequence to understand the static and dynamic aspects of genomes within the biological systems. Technologies are used to define sequence, sequence variation and gene expression. In addition, genomic tools can be used to manipulate genetic sequence and gene expression to understand the biological systems. Different tools are used to understand different levels of gene expression. Here we discuss about human leukocyte antigen (HLA) [7, 8, 11].

Human leukocyte antigen (HLA) is the most studied human gene in immunology. It is the most polymorphic gene in the genome with thousands of allelic variants with specificity for antigen recognition. Accurate assignment of HLA genotype is a requisite for certain bone marrow or organ transplantation. Accurate assignment of HLA genotype is required for certain bone marrow or organ transplantation. Serological HLA typing was used previously for donor matching. However, recently, this has been upgraded to high resolution HLA typing that is able to provide improved donor matching process and increased survival in recipients. Technological platform that has been used for such improvement is the deep sequencing method, which is a cost effective technique in clinical settings and can be used for multiple purposes. These include (i) identification of immunogenetic risk factor for disease; (ii) examine HLA polymorphism across population and pathogenic diversity and (iii) selection of immunodominmant HLA-restricted T cell epitopes to design vaccines. DNA sequencing technologies are also used to monitor immune responses to vaccines and profiling of T cell antigen receptor (TCR) or antibody repertoires. A general computational strategy for antibody repertoire analysis involves alignment, clustering and phylogenetic tree construction. Software such as MiTCR (Table 3) is used for efficient processing and analyzing of TCR sequences from millions of raw sequencing data generated from high throughput sequencing platforms. Repertoire analysis relies on having good reference sequence for proper statistical analysis, comparison and estimation of diversity. ImMunoGeneTics (IMGT) is the largest database of reference sequence for immunoglobulins, TCRs and MHCs. This database provides a web portal for researchers to compare upto 450,000 of their measured sequences against a reference sequence that enables detection of germ-line rearrangements identification of specific clones that might be associated with the disease [7,8,10, 11].

DNA sequencing technologies are also used to monitor human immune system in the context of population response to vaccines, profiling of T cell antigen receptor (TCR) or antibody repertoires. A general computational strategy for repertoire analysis involves alignment, clustering and phylogenetic tree construction. These require the use of special software such as MiTCR (Table **3**), which can efficiently process and analyze TCR sequences from millions of raw high-throughput sequencing reads. Repertoire analysis relies on having good reference sequence for proper statistical analysis for comparison and diversity estimates. ImMunoGeneTics (IMGT) information database contains the largest collection of reference sequence for immunoglobulins, TCRs, MHCs. This database provides a web portal for researchers to compare upto 450,000 of their measured sequences against a reference sequence to enable germ-line rearrangements and identify specific clones that might be associated with the disease [10].

Transcriptomics

Transcriptomics is the study of mRNA transcripts produced in a cell or tissue in response to a defined condition which can either be a diseased condition or normal cellular function. The mRNA levels in a cell are highly dynamic, with turnover time in the range of minutes to days. Investigation of the genome-wide patterns of mRNA expression in cells enables identification of the drivers of immune response such as cytokines, antigens and small molecules within cells and across organisms. Since RNA synthesis is a central process of the flow of genetic information in both eukaryotic and prokaryotic system. Isolated RNAs are therefore used for analytical and diagnostic purposes [7, 8, 11].

Different technologies have been used to measure the transcript levels in cells. cDNA microarray is the most popular method to measure whole-genome mRNA transcripts. However, in recent years, next generation sequencing technologies offered more benefits than microarrays. For example, RNA-Seq does not require knowledge of the sequence and can be used for the identification of RNA-editing events, novel exon and allele-specific differences [7]. It is also a powerful method to quantify transcriptomes and identify splice variants. By applying this method in the field of immunology, it has been possible to reveal the transcriptional profiles of B cells, monocytes, genetic reprogramming underlying the development of helper T cells, Th17 cell lineage entry and dendritic cell maturation in response to stimulators. Several software packages are available to perform differential gene expression analysis using RNA-seq. These tools are used to normalize RNA count data, identify differentially expressed genes and estimate false recovery rates. Other soft-wares such as Cufflinks and DEXSeq test are used for differential exon expressions to examine splice variants. ERANGE is used to analyze single neucleotide polymorphisms (SNPs) (Table **3**) [10].

In addition to transcriptional studies, another approach to understand and relate the genetic drivers of a disease is to measure DNA variation and transcriptional profiles from the same sample followed by statistical relationship between DNA variation and gene expression traits. Expression quantitative trait loci (eQTL) analysis is a robust statistical technique, which is used to compare variation in a quantitative trait (for example mRNA expression) to DNA variation at specific genomic loci. Although eQTL relationship suggests regulatory interaction between DNA-RNA (transcripts to SNP), genome wide analysis requires computationally intensive and efficient tools. MatrixEQTL is such a software package which can be used for efficient mathematical operations in modern computer programs with 2-3 orders of magnitude faster running time over other softwares [10].

In addition to eQTL analysis, another means of understanding immunological process and understanding drivers of disease are by system-wide genetic (GWAS) profiling [2, 12]. Genome wide measurements using protein-DNA interactions measured by chromatin immunoprecipitation (ChIP) and analyzed by DNA microarrays are used to correlate DNA transcription factor-binding sites with gene expression. However, more recently, genome wide association studies (GWAS) integrate omics datasets. More specifically, GWAS is the study of genetic variants among individuals and correlation with traits, such as disease susceptibility or drug responsiveness. Over 38 million single nucleotide polymorph- isms (SNPs) have been identified from the 1000 Genomes Project [7]. Another type of transcript is miRNA. These are non-coding small RNA molecules that act as transcriptional regulators of gene expression. Interestingly, individual miRNAs might have multiple targets and individual gene might be regulated by multiple miRNAs. The mechanisms of their regulation can be measured by microarray or gene sequencing technologies (Table **1**) [7]. Other type of transcriptional regulation occurs at the protein level. Techniques used to detect these regulations include hybridization of microarrays that probe entire genomic regions with chromatin immunoprecipitation (ChIP) products. Thus, it provides a high throughput method (ChIP-chip) to quantify the network of protein-DNA interactions. This technique has been used to determine the NF-kB binding sites in epithelial cells that are derived from human cervical cancer as well as binding sites for cMyc and p53 in human T cell lymphoma derived cell lines and human colorectal cancer derived cell line [7].

Proteomics

Proteins are the primary functional units of signalling pathways. Proteomics involves the measurement of expressed proteins in a given system and these are directly connected to pathway signalling molecules. Proteomic technologies include mass spectrometry (MS)-based and immuno-based methods, including protein microarrays. Another technology is mass cytometry, which uses transition element-tagged antibodies in flow cytometry and can be used tomeasure 40 parameter per cell. Another approach that is used in cancer research is tissue microarray (TMA), which consists of paraffin blocks where tissues from biopsy samples from different cancer patients are collected. The arrays consist of upto 1000 separate tissue cores and are assembled in an array fashion to allow multiplex histological analysis [7, 8, 11].

One drawback of proteomics study is that no technology is available to accurately measure the proteins in a system. Another drawback is that proteins are subject to post-translational modifications. As a result, many proteins remain undetected using the standard proteomics technologies. Posttranslational modifications include cleavage, acetylation, glycosylation, methylation, phosphorylation, SUMOylation and ubiquitination, all of which can impact protein function such as ligand binding, cellular location or even the prtoien half-life [7, 8, 11].

Phosphoproteomics is another branch of study of proteomics. Protein phosphorylation is a key regulator of signalling pathways but is transient in nature and can impact pathway dynamics in a complex way. Phosphoproteins can generate switch-like behavior in pathway signalling. Methods that have been used to quantify phosphoprotiens include MS-based and immune-based approaches. Databases that are cataloging post-translational modifications include PTMcode, PhosphoSitePlus and phosphELM (Table **1**) [7, 8, 11].

Metabolomics

Metabolomics is the study of the metabolites that are generated extracellularly or intracellularly in a cell or system. Different techniques that are used to measure metabolites include chromatographic or electrophoretic based MS and nuclear magnetic resonance spectroscopy (NMR). The human metabolome database (HMDB) contains more than 40000 annotated metabolites [7].

Metabolomics has been used for the discovery of biomarkers in several clinical settings, such as different types of cancer and has been used to understand the perturbed phenotypes when combined with proteomics and transcriptomics data [7].

One drawback of the metabolomics is that the concentration of the metabolites may vary from sample to sample or from one disease state to another. Metabolite concentrations reflect the function of the gene under a perturbed condition. Since the level of the intracellular or extracellular metabolites varies and often requires optimization of the technique in the laboratory setup, a robust tool to measure the exact level of metabolites is metabolic flux analysis (MFA). However, there is limited information on the application of this platform in immunotherapy and should be considered for model development implementing MFA with other HT platforms [7].

Computational Analysis

Computational tools are used to analyze high-throughput data and visualization of the large dataset for predictive model development. The HT technologies generate large datasets, which are considered as the bottleneck of the approach and are thought to mask the underlying cause of a disease or treated condition. To reduce the complexity of data mining and integrate data from different platforms, a number of analytical methods have been developed (Table **3**). For multivariate datasets, grouping or filtering can be applied based on statistical or mathematical features (such as clustering or factor analysis) [7].

For example, mRNA expression data have been used to build interaction networks to help understand pathway regulation. Clustering genes according to similar transcript profiles have been used to build co-expression networks. This method involves generation of a matrix of pair-wise correlation across samples where information on experimental systems, individuals, time series *etc.* is provided. The matrix is transferred into graphical representation in which the distance between genes (also known as nodes) is inversely related to the degree of correlation [7, 13].

Other useful methods for model construction include integration and combination of omics data with external information. Gene-set enrichment analysis is a standard method for transcriptome data analysis. It measures the enrichment for a group of genes, which belongs to a particular pathway or functional category based on gene ontology (GO) or Kyoto Encyclopedia of Genes and Genome (KEGG) annotations. Another popular method is Connectivity Map (cmap) approach, which uses pre-specified gene signatures to analyze transcript profiles [7, 13].

Graphical network models help in developing hypothesis generation where the network can be derived from mathematical relations, sematic relations or physical relations. Integrating multiple data type can provide a more complete picture of a system and reveals regulatory loops. Protein interaction data are employed to construct network scaffolds. Protein-protein interaction databases are useful for this purpose (Table **3**) [7].

Casual network modeling uses a large collection of biological cause and effect statements. Reverse causal analysis can be applied to identify network components upstream of the observed component with a differentially expressed gene [7].

Recently, systems biology has focused on integrating data from multiple omics technologies to help build predictive network models. This includes pathway topology, metabolic network and protein-DNA interaction information and genome-wide association studies (GWAS) [7, 13].

Pathway topology information includes information about genes with respect to the position of their gene products along a pathway and the relation of transcription factors and target gene products. This information is available from databases such as NCI pathway Interaction Database (PID), KEGG *etc.* These pathways are constructed using information from published literature and are curated by experts. More sophisticated methods include signaling pathway impact analysis (SPIA), probabilistic graphical models and Bayesian pathway analysis (BPA), incorporate pathway topology (might need to write more if time available) [7]. Another type of dataset used to understand targets and disease pathways is Gene Expression Omnibus (GEO) database. It connects disease concepts and combines protein-protein interaction data [7]. For network modeling or mathematical interpretation and modeling, specialized web-based tools are available for investigators to query, retrieve and analyze data from the available database at public repository. These are also known as bioinformatics tools. These bioinformatics tools are used for data analysis and interconnected modules enable cancer researchers to access the Cancer Genome Anatomy Project (CGAP) data of National Cancer Institute (NCI) [7, 13].

The CGAP database includes cancer-relevant genes and SNPs, malignant tissues and chromosomal aberrations in cancer patients. CGAP also provides information regarding the differential expression of a given gene in normal, precancerous and cancerous tissues based on Serial Analysis of Gene Expression (SAGE), as well as RNA interference (RNAi) constructs that target cancer-related genes, and diagrams of biochemical pathways and protein complexes [7, 13]. In addition to cancer related databases, immunology related databases are available too (Table 3). Immunomics is the study of the immune system in response to pathogens or antigens which induces immune responses. For cancer related studies, tumor associated antigens (TAAs) are of importance as these are extensively used for diagnosis and treatment purposes. Publicly available Human Potential Tumor Associated Antigen (HPtaa) database contains TTAs that are identified by in silico computing or modeling. HPtaa contains microarray expression data, SAGE data from GEO and Unigene expression data and knowledge bases of CGAP [7, 13]. It is a web query interface which provides information on potential TAAs overexpressed in several cancer types. Another database that gives information on humoral or cellular response to TAAs is documented in Cancer Immune Database (CID). It also contains information of gene features, protein coding gene and subcellular location (membrane or secretory proteins) [13].

Another database that gives information on humoral or cellular response to TAAs is documented in Cancer Immune Database (CID). The Academy of Cancer Immunology supported by Ludwig Institute has established CID. The database has information on all the gene products against an immune response in cancer patients including serological results, microscope images and cytotoxic assays. In addition, information on the type of cancer, disease stage and time of sample collection is available.

Another mentionable database is cancer-testis (CT) antigen database. It is a curated repository of annotated and computationally predicted cancer-testis antigens database. It provides information on genes, verified splice variants, genomic locations, gene duplications and bibliographical references [13].

APPLICATION OF SYSTEMS BIOLOGY APPROACH IN CANCER IMMUNOTHERAPY

Proper designing of cancer immunotherapy drugs requires identification of biomarkers that correlate to the diseased state and determination on the interaction of the components in a variety of circumstances. Systems biology is gradually becoming an important component in immune response monitoring and discovery of pharamcodynamic biomarker. The approach has been used in (i) characterizing immune cells, (ii) understanding the diversity of antibody responses to epitope spread, (iii) investigation on the dynamics of T-cell clones and (iv) immune characteristics of the tumor microenvironment. Earlier studies showed gene expression patterns associated with lymphocyte infiltration and tumor destruction following treatment with ipilimumab (CTLA-4 blockade). Further studies need to be performed to establish the post-treatment expression signatures to be used as biomarkers of overall survival rate upon ipilimumab therapy [2].

Discovery of New Targets

Therapeutic targets for cancer immunotherapy can be of two types (i) those that are expressed on the cells of the immune cells and (ii) antigens that are expressed by the tumor cells [10].

Under natural condition, antibody development against specific antigens is restricted to clonal selection. However, the range of the tumor antigens is wide and can be targeted by small molecules or monoclonal antibody therapies. The selection of the suitable tumor antigen is critical to develop an antigen-targeting cancer immunotherapy. These targets are expected to possess a number of attributes such as tumor or tissue specific alterations and immunogenicity. Off-target immunotherapies are more prone to have severe and difficult to control properties. Therefore, tumor or tissue specific antigens are particularly important. Some antigens such as KRAS, p53 and Her/neu that are used in immunotherapy are mutated or over-expressed [10].

Another group of immunotherapy drug target antigens shows restricted normal expression in certain tumors (*e.g.* the cancer testis antigens). In addition, tissue specific antigens such as gp100 for melanocytes, PAP or PSA for the prostate and CD19 for B cells have also been used effectively as targets for treating malignancies originating from those tissues. As antigens should have tumor or tissue specific alterations, the mining of gene expression or mutation databases and use of deep sequencing platforms have contributed to the discovery of many tumor antigens over the past several years [10].

In addition to selection of the correct antigen, immunogenicity is another critical consideration for selecting tumor antigen. Immunity against a tumor antigen depends on the recognition of the peptides from an antigen presented to the lymphocytes by the MHC molecules on the tumor cells as well as the professional antigen presenting cells (APCs). Immunogenicity can be assessed by (i) the frequency with which the antigen peptides are presented by the MHCs and (ii) the frequency with which naturally occurring cellular or humoral antigens are observed. Both experimental and computational methods can be used to assess immunogenicity. For example, high-throughput humoral profiling techniques can be used to detect antibodies. High-content protein microarrays are an alternative approach for the identification of antibodies against tumor antigens. Advantage of this technique is that antibodies against hundreds or thousands of self-antigens can be quantified rapidly using these microarrays. Moreover, MHC-restricted epitopes can be identified by computational predictions. Although SEREX is a productive approach, it is a laborious technique and may not yield quantitative data [5, 10]. However, computational predictions can be challenging because of their high degree of heterogeneity in length and sites of natural truncations. Therefore, mass spectrometry has been used as an experimental approach to identify and quantify the peptide epitopes from MHC-peptide complexes [7].

Understanding Therapeutic Mechanism of Action (MoA)

The molecular pathways involved in tumor surveillance and tumor escape mechanism are complex. By using the highthrouput omics platform, it is possible to understand the mechanisms leading to such events in the tumor micro-environment. Here we describe how omics platforms can be used to understand such changes in the contest of cancer immuno-therapies.

Transcriptional profiling using DNA microarray has been used to interrogate cellular pathways and investigate MoA in numerous studies. The technique has been used to characterize gene sets or signature molecules associated with immune cell lineages and activation and differentiation of signalling pathways (*e.g.*, T cell signalling, B-cell signalling, cytokine signalling *etc.*). These gene sets are a key to the interpretation of the new transcriptomic data derived from complex biological samples such as peripheral blood mononuclear cells (PBMC) or whole blood [7].

There are several ways to interpret a novel whole-genome gene expression data-set. This can be achieved either by using information from known biological pathways or gene sets derived from previous studies. The approach is also known as gene-set enrichment analysis. There are well curated databases for gene-sets or signatures (*e.g.*, MsigDB, PAGED and GeneSigDB) and biological pathways (*e.g.*, Gene Ontology, KEGG and Reactome). In addition, there are repositories of raw transcriptomic data from which gene sets can be derived (*e.g.*, gene expression omnibus or GEO). A number of statistical methods are available for determining enrichment which assess the genes from a previously known gene-set or pathawy and are significantly over-represented amongst a list of genes identified from a new experiemnt that is being analyzed. Despite its usefulness and widespread use, there are some limitations of gene-set based analyses for understanding MoA. For *e.g.*, gene sets are frequently incomplete and context dependent (*e.g.*, tissue or cell type specific). Since the quality of the gene sets determines the success of the approaches, incomplete or context specific gene-sets can be misleading to infer the mechanism of action (MoA) [3, 10].

Here we highlight a few examples of the application of expression profiling and data interpretation for the mechanistic characterization of cancer immuno-therapies.

DC or APC therapies are one type of cellular immunotherapy. Detailed characterizations of these cellular products are of particular importance to use them for therapy purposes. Gene-expression profiling can be used to characterize the activity and potency of these products [7].

DCs used for therapeutic applications are generated through culture with a wide range of activating factors such as cytokines, adjuvants *etc*. Depending on the nature of the cytokines or adjuvants used in their production, DCs have different properties. For example, DCs cultured with IFN-α-2β and GM-CSF to produce mature dendritic cells (DCAs) and GM-CSF and IL-4 to produce DC4 cells were compared using DNA microarrays. Comparison of mRNA profiles between DCA and DC4 revealed that the expression of genes involved in antigen presentation was increased in DCA relative to DC4. Increased expression was observed in TAP-2, HLA-DQ and HLA-DM. Up-regulation of TLRs, several TNF family ligands (*e.g.*, TRAIL, TNFα and Fas), and inflammatory chemokine receptors (*e.g.* CCR2) were identified that facilitated migration of DCs to the inflamed tissues. Consistent with the expression profiling, functional assays showed that DCAs were more potent mediators of naïve T-cell responses and tumor cell cytotoxicity than DC4 [7].

Global gene expression profiling of immature DCs matured with lipopolysaccharide (LPS, a TLR4 agonist), IFN-γ, IL-1β and TNF-α to evaluate different clinical DC maturation protocol extended the understanding of the association of particular genes and products of the pathway that are associated with clinical efficacy. This facilitated the development of reliable and effective production methods for cellular therapeutics as well as in establishing robust methods of quality control of these products [3, 7, 10].

Transcriptional profiling of complex and heterogeneous biological specimens along with bioinformatics methods for data interpretation significantly enabled the elucidation of the MoA associated with immunotherapeutic responses. Whole blood and PBMCs can be analyzed using transcriptional profiling and the data can be interpreted with gene sets. Whole blood and PBMC are also useful for phenotypic or functional characterization of the immune cells by conventional assays (such as multi-parameter flow-cytometry, cell proliferation or ELISpot). Gene-sets are associated with different immune cell-lineages, cell signalling pathways, cellular differentiation and activation (*e.g.*, naïve, memory and effector T cells or monocyte differentiation to macrophages and DCs). Although the computational methods are still under developement, progress in current methods is significantly beneficial to investigate *in vivo* MoA and clinical biomarkers using whole blood and PBMCs [3, 7, 10].

In addition to the above mentioned samples, transcriptomics profiling of tumors also provides insights into the *in vivo* MoA of cancer immunotherapies. Clinical studies from multiple cancer immunotherapy show evidence of increased lymphocyte infiltration within tumor samples. These are reflected by a higher expression of lymphocyte markers, cytokines and chemokines, which might be associated with better clinical outcome from the therapies. Pre-treatment of gene-expression signatures consisting of T-cell markers and cytokines from melanoma and non-small-cell lung tumor were found to be associated with overall survival upon treatment with MAGE-A3 vaccine in patients with tumors expressing the MAGE-A3 antigen. Studies with ipilimumab (an anti-CTLA-4 antibody) using gene-expression profiling of tumor biopsies collected from melanoma patients before and three weeks after the start of treatment in a Phase II clinical trial were reported. Transcriptional profiling of the pre-treatment tumors indicated that patients with high expression levels of immune related genes (T-cell activation, antigen presentation) were more likely to show clinical activity upon treatment with ipilimumab. Patients with clinical activity, ipilimumab treatment showed increased expression of genes involved in immune responses (IFN-γ-inducible genes and Th1-associated markers) and decreased the expression of melanoma antigens and cell-proliferation genes. These post-treatment gene expression changes were associated with the lymphocyte infiltrate into the tumors. Thus, gene expression profiling is providing valuable mechanistic insights into the *in vivo* activity of the immunotherapies against the tumor [3, 7, 10].

Assessment of Antigen Spread or Epitope Spread

An effective cancer immunotherapy which leads to the destruction of tumor tissue may lead to priming of T or B lymphocytes against tumor antigens that are not contained in the therapy. These antigens are known as secondary antigen and the phenomenon is referred to as antigen spread, epitope spread or determinant spread. Immune response against a broad group of antigen may promote more efficient killing of the tumor cells. Antigen spread or epitope spread has been observed in response to PSA-targeting immunotherapy, CTLA-4 blockade in melanoma and prostate cancer, Her2/neu vaccination for breast cancer and MUC1 DC vaccination in renal cancer patients [7].

Evaluation of humoral response against a diverse set of self-antigens can be explored using the high content protein or peptide microarrays. This technique has been used for the detection and validation of post-therapy antibody response to tumor antigens. For example, PAK6 is a tumor antigen against which both humoral and CD4+ T cell responses were observed post CTLA-4 blockade in prostate cancer patient. Immunization with PAK6 was protective in mouse tumor models. These observations indicate the future application of high-throughput technologies to study the breadth of the immune response to assess the therapeutic activity against the tumor *in vivo* [7].

Lymphocyte Receptor Sequencing and Monitoring of T-cell clones

High -throughput (HT) next generation technologies (NGS) have been applied to sequence and quantify antigen receptors on T and B lymphocytes. While antigen receptor molecules from certain B cells are secreted as antibodies and these are identified by using protein or peptide microarrays, NGS technologies have been applied to assess the diversity of receptors on the T cells that are specifically expressed on the T cell surface. Somatic recombination and addition or subtraction of nucleotides at the recombination junctions of T cell receptor generate a wide array of T cells with specificities against a wide array of antigens High-throughput DNA and RNA sequencing technologies allow deeper assessment of the T cell diversity. Sequencing of TCR (TCR-sequencing) can help to describe the dynamics of the T-cell repertoire before and after therapy and may aid in characterizing the efficacy of specific T- cell clones *in vivo* [7].

Biomarker Identification

Tumor gene expression profiling has been used to identify diagnostic marker in tumor samples and some are already in use in clinical practice. Ideal diagnostic markers or biomarkers are expected to have some properties such as readily detectable in body fluids, suitable for quantitative analysis, associated with relevant clinical outcomes, *e.g.*, survival, and indicative of the *in vivo* mode of action. The biomarkers can be predictive biomarkers related to pre-treatment or pharmacodynamic markers of post-treatment of clinical outcome [2, 3].

Therapeutic Biomarkers in the Tumor Environment

Tumor gene expression profile prior to any treatment is indicative of host immune response to the tumor. Tumor cells are resistant to attack for several reasons. These include expression of proteins that are anti-apoptotic, increased production of growth factors which support tumor growth, mutation in enzymes that lead to increased metabolic activity, secretion of immunosuppressive compounds and molecules by tumor associated macrophages, immature tumor-associated DCs (TADCs), Treg cells, IL-10 producing regulatory B cells, MDSCs and tumor cells themselves. Higher expressions of PDL1 by tumor immune filtrates and CTLA-4 and CX3CL1 are used to predict responses to PD-1 or PDL-1 specific treatment in several types of tumor including bladder cancer, NSCLC, melanoma and renal cell carcinoma. Expression of interferon-γ (IFNγ) secreted by tumor-specific T cells also indicates an ongoing immune response [2, 3].

T-helper cell activation and signaling pathways (iCOS-iCOSL and CD28 signaling) were found to be associated with prognosis. IHC and genetic profiling of tumor cells have been used to categorize cancer and treat them rationally. This categorization is based on the immunosuppressive mechanisms of the transformed cells [3]. Multiple groups have reported the discovery and validation of gene expression signatures from whole blood that are prognostic of overall survival in castrate-resistant prostate cancer. Profiling of whole blood or PBMC also provides predictive response to immunotherapies [2, 3].

By applying systems biology approaches and integrating data analysis from different platforms, a significant number of tumor antigens have been identified. We already mentioned some of the tumor antigens in chapter 1. With the advent of protein microarrays, it is now possible to identify tumor antigens with detectable serum antibodies. The method involves identification of immunogenic antigen peptides by combining tumor gene expression profiling data with mass spectrometric identification of MHC-restricted peptides from tumor specimens. These peptides were used to develop vaccines that are under clinical investigation [3].

In addition, tumor progression in patients can be detected by using multiple tumor antigens. The use of deep sequencing technologies can be used to survey the mutational profile of tumor antigens in an individual and this profile may be used to enable the formulation of individualized immunotherapies [7].

SNPs and other DNA variations can be useful as predictive markers. DNA variations are easier to assess compared to RNA as biological material since DNA is more stable compared to RNA and the number of variables can be limited *e.g.,* SNPs, which represent somatic mutation. At present, genome-wide studies in association with SNPs to clinical immunotherapy are lacking. However, SNP platforms that are focused on genes with known immune functions may provide a cost-effective way to perform large-scale genotyping studies in immunotherapy trials. In addition, integration of SNP data with other molecular studies associated with gene expression can significantly enhance the identification and annotation of functional SNPs associated with clinical outcomes. This approach will enable completion and evaluation of SNP association with clinical efficacy as well as validation of earlier results [2, 3, 5, 7].

Biomarkers of Post-treatment

These are also known as pharmacodynamic markers. Robust and reliable pharmacodynamic markers of clinical efficacy are a critical need in the development of cancer immunotherapy (need to paraphrase). Clinical outcome to cancer immunotherapy is not always reflected accurately by the conventional imaging measures for solid tumors. Tumor infiltration by active immune cells following therapy may be misleading as prolonged patient survival without reduced tumor progression can be observed [3, 7].

Immune response monitoring in clinical studies has traditionally been performed using techniques such as ELISA for measuring antibody levels, multiparameter flow cytometry for the characterization of cell phenotype, lymphocyte proliferation assays, ELISpot for quantitating antigen-specific cells and multiplexed cytokine/chemokine measurements [3, 7].

Protein microarrays were used in earlier studies for the high-throughput measurement of antibody responses post-therapy. In clinical studies, GVAX® (GM-CSF-secreting whole cell immunotherapy; Cell Genesys, CA, USA) was used to treat prostate cancer patient. Protein microarrays were used to identify specific antibody responses that were induced post-therapy. An antibody response against TARP (T cell alternative reading frame protein, a protein linked to prostate carcinogenesis) was significantly associated with the survival duration. Therefore, protein microarrays appear to be used for the discovery of post-treatment biomarkers of clinical outcome and can be translated for routine immune monitoring in patients [3, 7].

Model Validation

Systems biology can help in model validation. By identifying specific targeted and genetically altered characteristics in animal models, significant efforts are underway to develop more relevant animal models of human disease. Samples for biomarker studies are processed involving several steps. At first, samples are obtained using excisional or needle biopsy from patients. Tumor tissue is then processed either by enzymatic digestion followed by dimethyl sulfoxide freezing, by snap-freezing or by formaldehyde-fixation and paraffin-embedded (FFPE). The digested tumor material is then used to grow patient-derived xenografts (PDXs) in non-obese diabetic (NOD) mice that have severe combined immunodeficiency (SCID) and are deficient for the common delta-chain (IL-2RG). These tumor xenografts are then isolated to collect tumor infiltrating lymphocytes (TILs). TILS are then subject to flow cytometry studies or co-culture with tumor cell lines or used for adoptive transfer in PDX models [1].

Fresh tumor tissues are also processed to detect gene expression signatures by deep sequencing of whole-exome DNA or whole-exome RNA [1]. FFPE samples are analysed by immunohistochemistry (IHC). If matched blood samples are collected from patients with tumor source, the blood sample is processed by Ficoll density centrifugation for peripheral blood mononuclear cell (PBMC) isolation. PBMCs are used for flow cytometry analyses while serum samples are used for western blotting or protein detection. Results from these analyses are used to correlate patient outcomes to find predictive biomarkers [3].

In addition to model validation, animal models can be used to develop unbiased animal models of human disease. These are some novel applications of systems biology and can be used as quantitative model of human physiology. These models can serve several purposes such as (i) identification of key biological processes that affect disease progression and response to therapy, (ii) *in vivo* model analysis, (iii) simulation and analysis of cell-based assays to assess the predictive nature of the treatment and (iv) identification of methods to improve clinical relevance [3, 4].

Advancing Personalized Medicine

Systems biology approaches have been applied to personalized medicine to some extent. For example, there is genetic variation in normal *vs.* healthy human. Identification of single nucleotide polymorphisms (SNPs), or single-nucleotide DNA sequence variations in at least 1% population can affect our understanding of human physiology and disease. We already discussed approaches of systems biology that are used to identify biomarkers pre-treatment and post-treatment.

Clinicians can combine these approaches to personalized medicine. Systems biology approaches also provide systematic platforms that can be used effectively for the identification of clinical outcomes associated with efficacy or toxicity of the drug [3, 4].

Combination Therapy

Combination Therapy Systems biology has also been used in combination therapy . High throughput omics platforms of systems biology have been used to obtain information on the agents that can be used as immunotherapy drugs [3, 4]. In addition, biomarkers identified using the systems biology platforms can be used to develop algorithms that predict the probability of responses to immunotherapies. However, several drawbacks exist in this respect. For example, expression of PDL1 was partially lost in melanoma biopsy samples. This affected the partial predictive value in estimating the overall response rate and progression-free survival in patients who were treated with concomitant CTLA4 and PD1 blockade. Further studies of tumor samples at baseline and after treatment may help to prioritize optimal combinations provided that relevant targets are expressed. Adoption of non-invasive imaging techniques can be used to assess the immune filtrates [3, 4]. Another critical requirement for combination therapy is that there should be revisions of regulatory rules to evaluate the efficacy of the combinations in clinical trials. Considerations should be given to end-points that provide overall survival rates of the treatment. It also requires thorough investigation on the efficacy data of combination therapies. Importance should be given to the selection of combination partners such as (i) priming T cell responses by vaccines and adoptive T cell therapies directed to neoantigens that are presented by tumor cells, (ii) identify agents associated with immunogenic cell death; (iii) concomitant targeting of checkpoint inhibitors that are responsible for T cell anergy and/or exhaustion and (iv) delivery of artificial co-stimulatory and/or local pro- inflammatory agents. These therapeutic agents are expected to selectively target the tumor microenvironment and tumor-draining lymphoid tissue [3, 4].

CONCLUSION

Discovery and commercialization of an effective drug is a challenging process. Systems biology is a growing field in terms of technological developments particularly in genomics, transcriptomics, proteomics, metabolic flux analysis and computer simulation methods or software. Cancer immunotherapy is a growing field in terms of new therapy development, identification of new cancer antigens and immunomodulatory components that can be used for combination treatment. For example, monoclonal antibodies used for the treatment of cancer are one of the major contributions of tumor immunology to cancer patients. This success was built on integrating scientific research and technological advances in several fields of cancer immunology such as serological characterization of cancer cells, generation of antibodies targeting tumor antigens, exploration of the properties of antibodies *in vivo* and assessment of their function on cancer cells, detailed investigation on the signal transduction pathways related to cancer progression and an understanding of the complex interplay between cancer cells and the immune system.

However, major challenge in combining immunotherapies is that antibodies induce the immune systems whereas vaccines suppress the immune response [14]. During the clinical development phases, analyses are performed on the optimal trial design and discovery of biomarkers by integrating models of drugs and human patho-physiology [1]. The potential benefit of systems biology approach is that it provides comprehensive understanding of biological pathways, thereby providing information on the genetic cause of disease and its phenotypic interpretation. Furthermore, the information also facilitates de-risking or re-prioritizing therapeutic candidates in development in order to improve their probability of success in clinical testing. Regulatory agencies, such as US FDA, also encourage the application of such approaches, as these may improve and streamline the assessments of safety and effectiveness of the therapies. Indeed advances in research and clinical development of cancer immunotherapies with the application of systems biology tools have resulted in in depth understanding of the interplay between the immune system and tumor development. Some recent advances in this field have led to the regulatory approval of two therapies by the FDA. These are sipuleucel-T or Provenge ® and ipilimumab or Yervoy® . Some other immunotherapies that are currently under development and undergoing clinical testing are broadly classified into (i) vaccines or cellular immuno-therapies, (ii) cytokines and adjuvant therapies, (iii) immune-modulating antibodies and (iv) cancer vaccines containing tumor antigens [2, 3]. In conclusion, it can be stated that system biology is a robust approach in cancer immunotherapy and it can be applied at different stages of cancer immunotherapy development (Fig. **1**).

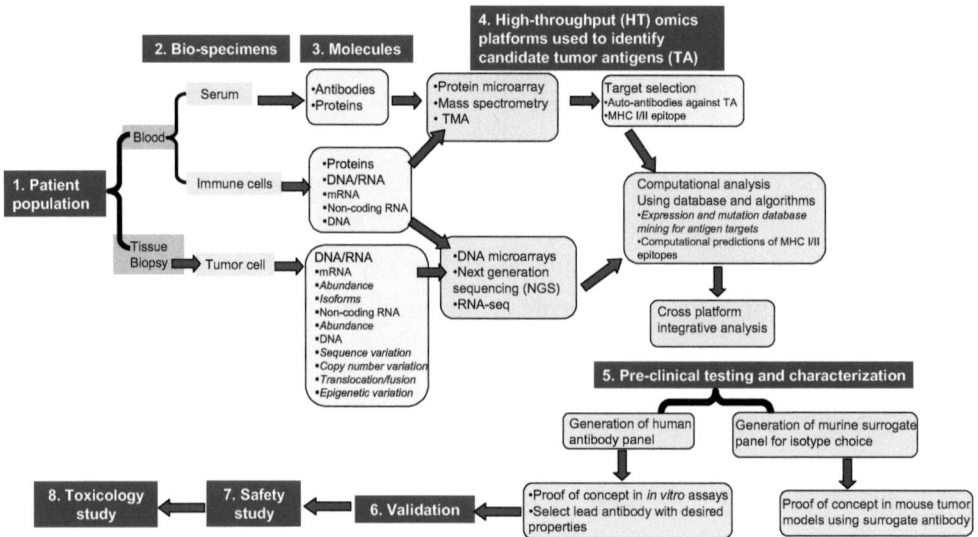

Fig. (1). Application of systems biology approaches in cancer immunotherapy.

CONFLICT OF INTEREST

The author confirms that author has no conflict of interest to declare for this publication.

ACKNOWLEDGEMENTS

Decleared none.

REFERENCES

[1]   Young DL, Michelson S. Future Outlook for Systems Biology. In: Young DL, Michelson S, Eds. Syst Biol Drug Discov Dev. 1st ed. New York City: Wiley & Sons, Inc. Publisher 2012; pp. 323-47.

[2]   Guhathakurta D, Sheikh NA, Meagher TC, Letarte S, Trager JB. Applications of systems biology in cancer immunotherapy: from target discovery to biomarkers of clinical outcome. Expert Rev Clin Pharmacol 2013; 6(4): 387-401.
[http://dx.doi.org/10.1586/17512433.2013.811814] [PMID: 23927667]

[3]   Melero I, Berman DM, Aznar MA, Korman AJ, Pérez Gracia JL, Haanen J. Evolving synergistic combinations of targeted immunotherapies to combat cancer. Nat Rev Cancer 2015; 15(8): 457-72.
[http://dx.doi.org/10.1038/nrc3973] [PMID: 26205340]

[4]   Simon R, Roychowdhury S. Implementing personalized cancer genomics in clinical trials. Nat Rev Drug Discov 2013; 12(5): 358-69.
[http://dx.doi.org/10.1038/nrd3979] [PMID: 23629504]

[5]   Ockert D, Schmitz M, Hampl M, Rieber EP. Advances in cancer immunotherapy Immunol Today 1999; 20(2): 63-5.
[PMID: 10098323]

[6]   Rahman M, Hasan MR. Cancer metabolism and drug resistance. Metabolites 2015; 5(4): 571-600.
[http://dx.doi.org/10.3390/metabo5040571] [PMID: 26437434]

[7]   Berg EL. Systems biology in drug discovery and development. Drug Discov Today 2014; 19(2): 113-25.
[http://dx.doi.org/10.1016/j.drudis.2013.10.003] [PMID: 24120892]

[8]   Shapira SD, Hacohen N. Systems biology approaches to dissect mammalian innate immunity. Curr Opin Immunol 2011; 23(1): 71-7.
[http://dx.doi.org/10.1016/j.coi.2010.10.022] [PMID: 21111589]

[9]   Ochsenbein AF. Principles of tumor immunosurveillance and implications for immunotherapy. Cancer Gene Ther 2002; 9(12): 1043-55.
[http://dx.doi.org/10.1038/sj.cgt.7700540] [PMID: 12522443]

[10]   Kidd BA, Peters LA, Schadt EE, Dudley JT. Unifying immunology with informatics and multiscale biology. Nat Immunol 2014; 15(2): 118-27.
[http://dx.doi.org/10.1038/ni.2787] [PMID: 24448569]

[11]   Charoentong P, Angelova M, Efremova M, *et al.* Bioinformatics for cancer immunology and immunotherapy. Cancer Immunol Immunother 2012; 61(11): 1885-903.
[http://dx.doi.org/10.1007/s00262-012-1354-x] [PMID: 22986455]

[12]   Smith KD, Bolouri H. Dissecting innate immune responses with the tools of systems biology. Curr Opin Immunol 2005; 17(1): 49-54.
[http://dx.doi.org/10.1016/j.coi.2004.11.005] [PMID: 15653310]

[13]   Pavlopoulou A, Spandidos DA, Michalopoulos I. Human cancer databases (review). Oncol Rep 2015; 33(1): 3-18. [review].
[http://dx.doi.org/10.3892/or.2014.3579] [PMID: 25369839]

[14]   Morgan AC, Foon KA. Monoclonal Antibody Therapy of Cancer : Preclinical Models and Investigations in Humans. Boston: Martinus Nijhoff 1986.

CHAPTER 6

Perspectives

Abstract: Both system biology and cancer immunotherapy are emerging fields in life sciences research. Immunotherapy is considered as targeted treatment modalities for cancer. However, the complex nature of the tumor environment affects the efficacy and clinical outcome of this type of therapy. Combination therapy can be a solution. But this requires investigation at the cellular and molecular level of effect of the drugs. Systems biology is such a powerful tool, which allows the cellular level understanding and has been used in target discovery and validation in different fields of cancer research. Despite this advantage, challenges exist in large dataset mining. In this concluding chapter, we discuss some of the challenges and possible future directions that may help to overcome this problem.

Keywords: Animal models, Cancer, Inflammation, Software tools, Systems biology, Targets, Validation.

INTRODUCTION

Cancer is caused from inflammation. As a result, tumor cells grow in the presence of heterogeneous cell population such as epithelial cells, vascular and lymphatic vessels, cytokines, chemokines and infiltrating immune cells. This heterogeneous cell population is at different stages of growth, differentiation and metabolic state. Therefore, design and development of drugs as anticancer agent is a challenging task for researchers and pharmaceutical companies and requires extensive knowledge on its surrounding environment to get the systems level understanding of the diseased and treated cells. Systems biology approach offers a robust tool to study the molecular and cellular level of a cell. Therefore, the purpose of this volume was to discuss the application of this approach in possible areas of cancer immunotherapy.

The presence of immune-surveillance system provides natural protection against cancer. However, few of the cancer cells carry mutation in genes of the anti-tumor immune response, which helps these cells in immune escape and immune evasion process (Chapter 1). Cancer cells are also known to hijack the body's normal cellular functions. A number of oncogenes and proto-oncogenes play important role in this process and aid in cancer progression involving different signalling molecules, transcription factors and cascades of protein molecule of the same signalling pathway (Chapter 2). Cancer cells also show deregulated metabolic pathways and these have been associated with drug resistance property. Interestingly, many cells of the anti-tumor immune response also show high proliferation and growth rate like the normal cells (Chapter 3). This creates non-specific effect on these antitumor cells when treated with anticancer drugs, especially chemotherapy drugs. Most of the conventional anticancer drugs are less specific and the side effects are enormous. Therefore, targeted therapies with less toxicity are of importance nowadays. Immunotherapy drugs are considered as targeted therapy and some of them received US FDA approval. However, immunotherapy drugs have also drawbacks as these are effective only on narrow range of cells. Therefore, combination therapies have been proposed at clinical and pre-clinical trials (Chapter 4).

Since its execution, systems biology and omics technologies have been widely used in the field of oncology and extensively used for characterizing the molecular complexity and heterogeneity of tumor not only for the development of targeted therapies but also for the identification of responder populations for such treatments (Chapter 5). In addition, the approach has been used for disease subtyping, disease progression and multi-gene diagnostic tests using gene expression profiling arrays [1 - 3]. Systems biology is also used in drug or target identification and validation and has been proposed for regulatory bodies to incorporate the modeling approach for drug approval policy. This process comprises of the complex set of experiments that aim to identify the key molecular drivers of disease and confirm the pharmacological modulation of the drug-in-development that leads to net clinical benefit. Thus, systems biology approaches can be used to enhance trial design, execution and analysis of drugs entering clinical studies.

However, challenges exist with large dataset mining of the omics platform. Several steps can be taken once the challenges are identified [4, 5]. In chapter 5, we discussed some of the challenges associated with the design of immunotherapy development. Here we extend our discussion on marketing of drugs and challenges associated with clinical trials.

CHALLENGES WITH MARKETING, CLINICAL TRIAL AND SAFETY ISSUE

Drug discovery and development companies are often need to make rapid and rational decision to place a product in the market in the face of incomplete clinical trial data. This was a significant concern when drug design and discovery groups were dependent on cell based reductionist approach and non-validated animal models on the human condition. Additional challenge is whether the drug should advance into phase III trial or not [6, 7].

The success rate of new drugs entering clinical studies is at historic low. The success rate of novel drugs also depends on the type of disease. Higher success rates are reported in infectious disease and cardiovascular disease whereas lower rates are reported for oncology and disease of the central nervous system. The most frequent cause of failure is lack of efficacy, particularly at the late stage of large scale pivotal studies. This significantly increased the cost for pharmaceutical companies leading to decreased rate of production of novel drugs. However, to enhance the efficacy and safety of drugs entering clinical trials, FDA approved model based drug development (MBDD) improved decision making and acquisition of knowledge from clinical studies This saved significant cost for pharmaceutical companies [4, 6, 8].

Challenges with novel drugs also exist during clinical trial and at several phases such as discovering the dose response in relation to the efficacy and toxicity of the drug, patient subgroups and validation stage. Model based data integration and analysis can improve our understanding of the clinical path and confirm processes. Since the systems approach integrates complex data on clinical studies such as disease process, time scale and clinical endpoints, previous information from other studies and heterogeneous clinical subjects, this improves quantitative modeling and facilitates rapid acquisition of knowledge of a drug in trial. Pharmaceutical companies, researchers and regulatory agencies can use these analytical approaches for comprehensive decision making on novel drugs [6].

Another challenge which is more specific to immunology is to determine baseline immunological states from molecular profiles and associate the molecular states with clinical outcome, *i.e.* the clinical phenotype. It was possible to make some progress through the integration of multiple data sources from medium sized cohorts, but challenges remain for bigger sample sizes from diverse demographic location to make clinically meaningful conclusions. Large scale consortia from different demographic locations can facilitate sample sizing and publicly available data repositories can provide another meaningful mechanism [9].

More challenges are observed in applying metabolic flux analysis (MFA), a part of metabolomics in cancer immunotherapy. This technique is used to understand the protein and enzyme level interaction within the cell where the reaction rates are dependent on the intracellular metabolite level. Although, this technique has been used to understand the drug resistance properties in cancer cells, in cancer immunotherapy, this is a very new technique and requires future attention as this is a robust tool that can be used to understand the phenotype of the diseased cell [1, 10].

FUTURE DIRECTIONS

By addressing the above challenges for new drug to be in market place, which is associated with patient outcome and large cohort study, and considering systems biology as a robust tool, several improvements are required in this approach.

Mining the large datasets generated from omics platforms requires people trained on computer simulation and modeling approaches. As a result, most of the data generated from the high-throughput platforms remain undetermined. Therefore, there is a need for tools that do not require specialized training so that researchers can easily analyze the large dataset for further assessment and integrate network models. This problem can be minimized by developing interactive software tools that will allow visualization of complex systems. Examples of such tools are Iris100 and Cytoscape [9]. The annotation tools allow network modeling of specific pathway or cell-type associations where genomics and proteomics networks can be viewed [11, 12]. Similar type of tools are required that will allow clicking on genes of interest for the synthesis of related literature and other forms of regulation such as epigenetic or miRNA-mediated changes. In addition, flexible network models generated from parent models that integrate molecular interactions with phenotypic or clinical data on medical records, histologic data and magnetic resonance images or other clinical images would be expected. In chapter 5, we discussed some of the bioinformatics tools that are used for the analysis of large datasets. However, more tools are under investigation. These are expected to provide accurate and comprehensive models of complex immune system dynamics and integrate multiple layers of profiling data.

CONFLICT OF INTEREST

The author confirms that he have no conflict of interest to declare for this publication.

ACKNOWLEDGEMENTS

Decleared none.

REFERENCES

[1] Rahman M, Hasan MR. Cancer metabolism and drug resistance. Metabolites 2015; 5(4): 571-600.
[http://dx.doi.org/10.3390/metabo5040571] [PMID: 26437434]

[2] Kalos M, June CH. Adoptive T cell transfer for cancer immunotherapy in the era of synthetic biology. Immunity 2013; 39(1): 49-60.
[http://dx.doi.org/10.1016/j.immuni.2013.07.002] [PMID: 23890063]

[3] Guhathakurta D, Sheikh NA, Meagher TC, Letarte S, Trager JB. Applications of systems biology in cancer immunotherapy: from target discovery to biomarkers of clinical outcome. Expert Rev Clin Pharmacol 2013; 6(4): 387-401.
[http://dx.doi.org/10.1586/17512433.2013.811814] [PMID: 23927667]

[4] Melero I, Berman DM, Aznar MA, Korman AJ, Pérez Gracia JL, Haanen J. Evolving synergistic combinations of targeted immunotherapies to combat cancer. Nat Rev Cancer 2015; 15(8): 457-72.
[http://dx.doi.org/10.1038/nrc3973] [PMID: 26205340]

[5] Kitano H. Systems Biology: A Brief Overview. Science 295: 1662-4.
[http://dx.doi.org/10.1126/science.1069492]

[6] Young DL, Michelson S. Future outlook for systems biology. In: Young DL, Michelson S, Eds. Syst

Biol Drug Discov Dev. 1st ed. New York City: Wiley & Sons, Inc. Publisher 2012; pp. 323-47.

[7]   Hernández Patiño CE, Jaime-Muñoz G, Resendis-Antonio O. Systems biology of cancer: moving toward the integrative study of the metabolic alterations in cancer cells. Front Physiol 2012; 3: 481.
[http://dx.doi.org/10.3389/fphys.2012.00481] [PMID: 23316163]

[8]   Hornberg JJ, Bruggeman FJ, Westerhoff HV, Lankelma J. Cancer: a systems biology disease. Biosystems 2006; 83(2-3): 81-90.
[http://dx.doi.org/10.1016/j.biosystems.2005.05.014] [PMID: 16426740]

[9]   Kidd BA, Peters LA, Schadt EE, Dudley JT. Unifying immunology with informatics and multiscale biology. Nat Immunol 2014; 15(2): 118-27.
[http://dx.doi.org/10.1038/ni.2787] [PMID: 24448569]

[10]   Mesure D. Cancer metabolic and immune reprogramming : the intimate Interaction between cancer cells and microenvironment. J Cancer Prev Curr Res 2014; 1: 1-8.

[11]   Charoentong P, Angelova M, Efremova M, *et al.* Bioinformatics for cancer immunology and immunotherapy. Cancer Immunol Immunother 2012; 61(11): 1885-903.
[http://dx.doi.org/10.1007/s00262-012-1354-x] [PMID: 22986455]

[12]   Ram PT, Mendelsohn J, Mills GB. Bioinformatics and systems biology. Mol Oncol 2012; 6(2): 147-54.
[http://dx.doi.org/10.1016/j.molonc.2012.01.008] [PMID: 22377422]

SUBJECT INDEX

A

Animal models   37, 124, 125, 143, 144, 149, 151

Apoptosis   20, 27, 29, 30, 32, 65, 69, 73, 85, 97, 101, 102, 111, 116

Arginine metabolism   42, 49, 51, 52, 67

Autophagy pathway   42, 81-83

B

Biomarkers   7, 132, 135, 136, 139, 141, 148, 153

C

Cancer   10, 11, 29, 47, 48, 50, 111, 131, 132, 152-154

Checkpoint blockades   86

Chemotherapy   11, 25, 37, 42, 77, 78, 86, 100, 102, 103, 113, 125, 150

Circulating tumor cells   3, 38, 41

Combination therapy   ii, 42, 86, 90, 92, 113, 118, 119, 122, 124, 125, 145, 149

Cytokines   3, 8, 10, 11, 13, 26, 33, 44, 46, 53, 55, 58, 59, 61, 62, 73, 74, 87, 91, 106, 120, 129, 138, 139, 147, 149

D

Dendritic cells   3, 6, 7, 9, 10, 19, 30, 33, 35, 40, 44, 46, 50, 54, 64, 69, 79, 92, 97, 98, 104, 106, 108, 121, 138

Drug discovery   122, 148, 151

I

Immune-metabolism   42

Immune-suppressors   42

Immune-surveillance   3, 7, 150

Immuno-escape   3, 30

Immuno-system   3

Immunotherapy

Immunotherapy   13, 39, 59, 84, 99, 100, 102, 108, 113, 115, 132, 135, 136, 142, 143, 145-154

Inflammation   ii, 3, 21, 30, 39, 40, 43, 45, 50, 53, 56, 70, 71, 73, 78, 84, 95, 118, 149

J

JAK-STAT   69, 71, 72, 84

L

Leptin   42, 44, 48, 49, 67

M

Monoclonal antibodies   86, 87, 93, 94, 97, 99, 102, 104, 109, 121, 146

Myc   37, 38, 62, 69, 71, 73, 76, 77, 81, 84

O

Omics platforms   ii, 122, 125, 126, 137, 145, 152

P

p53   14, 15, 24, 37, 58, 69, 77, 78, 83, 85, 115, 131, 136

Personalized medicine   95, 122, 123, 144, 145

R

Reactive oxygen species   11, 27, 35, 42, 44, 46, 66, 67, 78

Regulatory T cells   3, 9, 12, 18, 25, 36, 40, 47, 54, 93, 100, 109

S

Signal transduction pathways   61, 69, 80, 83, 146

Software tools   125, 149, 152

www.ingramcontent.com/pod-product-compliance
Lightning Source LLC
Chambersburg PA
CBHW041708210326
41598CB00007B/579